CLINICAL MANIFESTATIONS OF RESPIRATORY DISEASE

Second Edition

Clinical Manifestations of Respiratory Disease
Second Edition

TERRY DES JARDINS, M.Ed., R.R.T.
Department of Respiratory Therapy
Parkland College
Champaign, Illinois

YEAR BOOK MEDICAL PUBLISHERS, INC.
CHICAGO • LONDON • BOCA RATON • LITTLETON, MASS

A Year Book Medical Publishers imprint of Mosby-Year Book, Inc.

Mosby-Year Book, Inc., 11830 Westline Industrial Drive, St. Louis, MO 63146.

3   4   5   6   7   8   9   0   PC   94   93   92

Library of Congress Cataloging in Publication Data

Des Jardins, Terry R.
    Clinical manifestations of respiratory disease. 2nd ed.

    Bibliography: p.
    Includes index.
    1. Respiratory organs—Diseases.   I. Title.
RC731.D47   1990   616.2   90-2363
ISBN 0-8151-2432-5

Sponsoring Editor: Kevin M. Kelly
Associate Director, Manuscript Services: Frances M. Perveiler
Production Project Coordinator: Carol A. Reynolds
Proofroom Supervisor: Barbara M. Kelly

To Jane, Jennifer and Michelle, and to Uncle Jim and Janelle _____

To cease smoking is the easiest thing I ever did.
I ought to know because I've done it a thousand times.
Mark Twain

must have a large enough sampling fraction to make your sample representative of your research population. In practice, social science research often deals with a huge population in a city, a county, or a state, and the sample that the researchers can draw is often nothing as compared with the size of the total research population. In such cases, people often raise questions as to what is the use of the sample studies. Yet, as a matter of fact, statisticians have proved that for the study of any single variable, what counts in determining the sample size is not the sampling fraction, nor the size of the research population, but the variance of the variable, or the heterogeneity of the population in that particular aspect. No matter how large your research population is, the required minimum sample size is solely dependent on the variance of the focal variable for any given allowable error and confidence level when the sample statistic is used to represent the population parameter. In the case of a relational analysis, what counts is the magnitude of the association between variables (called the effect size). We will further discuss some of the terms and ideas later.

In statistics, the issue of determining the size of a random sample has been first related to the logic of statistical inference. Since the calculation of a test quantity is based on the size of the sample, it is very natural to transform the formula and derive the needed sample size in research design based on predetermined test condition. This logic, however, has been shown insufficient, since what can be determined in the formula is only part of the potential error called Type I error. There is another kind of error, called Type II error, that cannot be addressed by this traditional method. The two types of errors will be discussed in chapter eleven. In recent years, there has emerged a new and popular technique called the analysis of statistical power. Statistical power stands for the probability of correctly rejecting a null hypothesis in an empirical study. There are books as well as computer software now available for calculating statistical power and conducting detailed analysis. Like the people who would follow the vogue of their times, researchers nowadays are expected to present some sort of power analysis in almost every research proposal. But you should not feel too self-satisfied by just being able to deal with that requirement, even though it represents a real progress both in you and in science. What makes the matter complicated and the use of power analysis very limited is that the variance of any single variable and the effect size of any association between variables in the population are actually unknown. The estimates provided by merely one or a few pilot studies could be misleading. In addition, your study cases are usually comprised of a good number of variables; and those that constitute the real cases

PREFACE

This textbook is designed to provide the student with (1) an illustration of what each disease covered actually looks like in the lungs or, more specifically, how each disease anatomically alters the lungs; (2) a straightforward description of the cause, or etiology, of the disease; (3) an overview of the cardiopulmonary clinical manifestations associated with the disease and, just as important, the major known pathophysiologic mechanisms that may cause such clinical manifestations; (4) the general management of the disease; and (5) a set of self-assessment questions at the end of each chapter. This book is written primarily for respiratory care practitioners, critical care nurses, emergency room nurses, anesthetists, and medical students interested in pulmonary disorders.

The material in this textbook is based upon my personal experiences as an educator and instructor of both cardiopulmonary anatomy and physiology and respiratory pathology since 1973. In writing this textbook, I have striven to present a realistic balance between the esoteric language of pathophysiology and the simple, straight-to-the-point approach generally preferred by busy students.

Terry Des Jardins, M.Ed., R.R.T.

ACKNOWLEDGMENTS _____

Several individuals played important roles in the development of the second edition of this textbook. Again, my deepest thanks and appreciation go to Dr. Thomas DeKornfeld for the time he spent reading and editing drafts of the manuscript. Dr. DeKornfeld's constructive criticism regarding the medical, anatomic, physiologic, and pathophysiologic accuracy of the text, the environmental and structural format of the text, and the readability of the manuscript were crucial. For help in obtaining certain x-ray films reproduced in this text, I am grateful to Dr. Edward Didier and Dr. Joseph Rau. Finally, but certainly by no means least, I extend a very special thank-you to Carol Prusa, biomedical artist, for the wonderful artwork presented throughout this textbook. Ms. Prusa's artistic talents and perceptive insights are of superior quality.

Terry Des Jardins, M.Ed., R.R.T.

HOW TO USE THIS BOOK _____

Chapter 1 provides the reader with (1) the basic steps and skills involved in chest assessment, (2) the common clinical manifestations that recur from one respiratory disorder to another, and (3) the major known pathophysiologic mechanisms that cause the clinical manifestations presented in this section. In subsequent chapters on the various respiratory diseases, the student is often referred back to specific pages in Chapter 1 to supplement the identified clinical manifestations associated with the respiratory disease under discussion.

In preparing Chapter 1, I have endeavored to show the pathophysiologic mechanisms responsible for the following clinical manifestations:

- Common chest assessment findings
  - Tactile and vocal fremitus
  - Dull percussion note
  - Hyperresonant percussion note
  - Bronchial breath sounds
  - Diminished breath sounds
  - Crackles and rhonchi
  - Wheezing
  - Pleural friction rub
  - Whispered pectoriloquy
- Other common clinical manifestations
  - Cyanosis
  - Increased respiratory rate
  - Pulmonary function study findings in restrictive and obstructive disorders
  - Common abnormal arterial blood gas values seen in respiratory diseases
  - Increased heart rate, cardiac output, and blood pressure
  - Increased central venous pressure/decreased systemic blood pressure
  - Cough, sputum production, and hemoptysis
  - Use of the accessory muscles during inspiration
  - Use of the accessory muscles during expiration
  - Increased anteroposterior chest diameter (barrel chest)
  - Pursed-lip breathing
  - Polycythemia, cor pulmonale
  - Digital clubbing
  - Chest pain/decreased chest expansion
  - Substernal/intercostal retractions

Chapters 2 through 23 provide the reader with information on common respiratory diseases. Basically, each chapter on a specific respiratory disorder adheres to the following format: anatomic alterations of the lungs, etiology of the disease process, overview of the cardiopulmonary clinical manifestations, general management of the disorder, and a set of self-assessment questions.

ANATOMIC ALTERATIONS OF THE LUNGS

Each chapter on a respiratory disease begins with a detailed illustration showing the anatomic effects of the disease on the lungs. While serious efforts have been made to illustrate each disorder accurately in carbon dust at the beginning of each chapter, artistic license has been taken to emphasize certain anatomic points and pathologic processes.* The subsequent text in each chapter discusses the disease in terms of (1) the anatomic alterations illustrated in the figure; (2) the pathophysiologic mechanisms activated throughout the respiratory system as a result of the anatomic alterations; (3) the clinical manifestations that develop in response to the pathophysiologic mechanisms; and (4) the basic respiratory therapy modalities used to improve the anatomic alterations, pathophysiologic mechanisms, and the clinical manifestations activated by the disease.

ETIOLOGY

A discussion of the etiology of the disease follows the presentation of anatomic alterations of the lungs. When appropriate, illustrations are included in this section.

OVERVIEW OF THE CARDIOPULMONARY CLINICAL MANIFESTATIONS ASSOCIATED WITH THE DISORDER

An overview of the major cardiopulmonary clinical manifestations associated with the disorder follows the section on etiology. This section represents the central theme of this text. Many clinical manifestations associated with the disorder refer the reader back to specific pages in Chapter 1 for a broader discussion of the pathophysiologic mechanisms responsible for the identified sign or symptom. When a particular clinical manifestation is unique to the respiratory disorder under discussion (e.g., x-ray findings), however, the pathophysiologic mechanisms responsible for the sign or symptom and related clinical information are presented in this section.

Not every sign or symptom that may be associated with a particular pulmonary disorder is included in the clinical manifestation section, nor does this section attempt to present the "absolute" pathophysiologic bases for development of any clinical manifestation. Only the more prominent cardiopulmonary clinical manifestations are discussed. The student is also cautioned that the clinical manifestations presented in this text are only based on the respiratory disorder under discussion. In the clinical setting, the patient often has a combination of respiratory problems—emphysema compromised by pneumonia, for example. When such a condition exists, the patient will likely present clinical manifestations related to both pulmonary disorders.

*Chapter 23, Sleep Apnea, presents a line illustration at the beginning of the chapter.

GENERAL MANAGEMENT OR TREATMENT OF THE DISEASE

Each chapter provides a brief overview of the general management or treatment of the disease. It is not the intent of this text to provide a comprehensive section concerning the management or treatment of respiratory disorders. Several excellent textbooks dealing with this subject matter already exist. A general overview of the more common therapeutic modalities used in treating a particular disorder are discussed.

It should be stressed that while several respiratory therapy modalities may be safe and effective in treating a respiratory disorder, the respiratory care practitioner must have a clear conception of how the therapies work to offset the anatomic alterations of the lungs, the pathophysiologic mechanisms, and the clinical manifestations activated by the disease. Without such understanding, the respiratory therapist merely goes through the motions of administering the therapy, with the result that the safety and effectiveness of the therapy may be jeopardized.

SELF-ASSESSMENT QUESTIONS

Each respiratory disease chapter concludes with a set of self-assessment questions. The student may be asked questions that are directly related to the material presented in the respiratory disease chapter, the pathophysiologic mechanisms (which are presented in Chapter 1) that may be responsible for the common clinical manifestations associated with the disease, or the general management of the disease, which may include related information from the appendixes.

GLOSSARY AND APPENDIX

Finally, a glossary and an appendix are provided at the end of the text. The Appendix includes the following:

- A table of symbols and abbreviations commonly used in respiratory physiology
- Medications used in treatment of cardiopulmonary disorders, including
  - Sympathomimetic agents
  - Parasympatholytic (anticholinergic) agents
  - Xanthine bronchodilators
  - Corticosteroids
  - Mucus-controlling agents
  - Expectorants
  - Antibiotic agents
  - Positive inotropic agents
  - Diuretics
- Techniques used to mobilize bronchial secretions
- Hyperinflation techniques
- The ideal alveolar gas equation
- Physiologic dead space calculation
- Units of measurement
- Mathematical discussion of Poiseuille's law
- Answers to the self-assessment questions

CONTENTS _____

in the population could be countless. It is unlikely that you are able to conduct power analysis beforehand for every variable and every relation that will turn out to be important in later data analysis. Moreover, if you employ more complex procedures than simple random sampling in your study, the calculation of statistical power and required sample size for just one variable or association could be a very demanding task.

The usual practice, therefore, is to apply the mathematical formula only to the most important variable(s) and association(s), or the variable(s) of largest range of variation and the association of least effect size in a study. And the results are only to be taken as a reference. In making the final decision, your resources, especially available funding, will play an important part. The rule of thumb is to study as many cases as you can afford, since a larger sample size will help reduce the chance of error and increase the statistical confidence. The size of the population does not make much difference as long as you can maintain good randomness in drawing your samples. The use of various statistical techniques, especially statistical control, also demands large sample size. And the requirement cannot be exactly calculated because data analysis needs vary from time to time. If your sample size is less than thirty ($N<30$), you may need some special treatment in applying certain statistical procedures. Some experts would advise you to try to get a random sample of at least 100 cases; others might suggest you to get even more if at all possible. If you have a random sample sized several hundred or over a thousand, you will probably have enough statistical power to perform most of the statistical analyses. Generally speaking, samples employed in social science research tend to be relatively large. While smaller samples may be enough for a natural science study including the biological investigation of human beings, larger samples are usually required of social or psychosocial research because of the huge differences in human behavioral and social lives.

Large size alone, however, does not guarantee that you will capture all the qualitative features and characteristics of your research population. Another way to increase the representativeness of your sample is to stratify a heterogeneous population before you apply either simple random sampling or systematic sampling. This is called stratified random sampling, which can reduce the sampling error and increase the effectiveness by minimizing within-stratum differences while maximizing the between-stratum differences. One of the two basic random sampling procedures discussed above can then be applied to each stratum by using the same or different sampling proportions. When you use

CLINICAL MANIFESTATIONS OF RESPIRATORY DISEASE

Second Edition

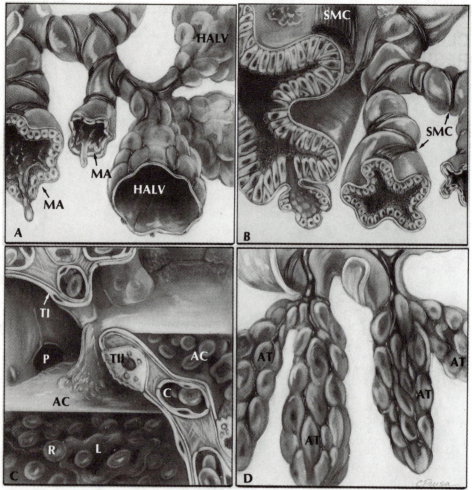

DISEASED LUNG

FIG 1–1.
Diseased lung. **A,** tracheobronchial inflammation accompanied by mucus filling and air trapping. **B,** bronchial smooth constriction accompanied by air trapping. **C,** alveolar consolidation. **D,** atelectasis. *MA* = mucus accumulation; *HALV* = hyperinflated alveoli; *SMC* = smooth muscle constriction; *TI* = type I cell; *TII* = type II cell; *P* = pores of Kohn; *AC* = alveolar consolidation; *C* = capillaries; *R* = red blood cells; *L* = lymphocytes; *AT* = atelectasis.

CHEST ASSESSMENT AND COMMON CLINICAL MANIFESTATIONS OF RESPIRATORY DISEASES

When the lungs are affected by disease or trauma, they are anatomically altered to some degree, depending on the severity of the injury. In general, the anatomic alterations caused by an injury can be classified as either an *obstructive lung disorder*, a *restrictive lung disorder*, or a *combination of both*. Figure 1–1,A and B illustrate some anatomic alterations that lead to an obstructive lung disorder. Figure 1–1,C and D illustrate some anatomic alterations that lead to a restrictive lung disorder. Table 1–1 lists some common respiratory diseases and their general classification.

When the *normal anatomy* of the lungs is altered, certain *pathophysiologic mechanisms* throughout the respiratory system are activated. These pathophysiologic mechanisms in turn cause various *clinical manifestations* that can be readily identified in the clinical setting (e.g., an increased heart rate, a depressed diaphragm, or an elevated functional residual capacity). In view of this relationship, the respiratory care practitioner must first have a basic knowledge of (1) the anatomic alterations of the lungs that are caused by the disease, (2) the possible pathophysiologic mechanisms activated by the disease, and (3) the various clinical manifestations associated with the disorder.

To identify the anatomic alterations of the lungs, pathophysiologic mechanisms, and clinical manifestations associated with a respiratory disorder, a general physical examination of the chest should first be conducted.

CHEST ASSESSMENT

The physical examination of the chest and lungs should be performed in an orderly and consistent fashion. The typical sequence is as follows:

- Inspection
- Palpation
- Percussion
- Auscultation

TABLE 1–1.
General Respiratory Disease Classifications

Respiratory Disorder	Obstructive	Restrictive	Combination
Chronic bronchitis	X		
Emphysema	X		
Asthma	X		
Bronchiectasis*			X
Cystic fibrosis*			X
Pneumoconiosis			X
Pneumonia		X	
Pulmonary edema		X	
Adult respiratory distress syndrome		X	
Flail chest		X	
Pneumothorax		X	
Pleural diseases		X	
Kyphoscoliosis		X	
Tuberculosis		X	
Fungal diseases		X	
Idiopathic (infant) respiratory distress syndrome		X	

*Most commonly seen as an obstructive lung disorder.

Inspection

The examiner may obtain a large amount of important information by inspecting the chest and confirming the presence or absence of certain clinical features. A significant amount of information can be gathered that has gone unrecognized by the patient. During inspection, the examiner should particularly note the following:

- Whether the patient is short of breath while talking. Does the patient stop to breathe after speaking only a few words?
- The use of accessory muscles during inspiration or expiration.
- The patient's posture while sitting. Individuals in respiratory distress often lean forward when seated, hold on to a stationary object, and hunch their shoulders forward.
- The patient's ventilatory pattern (rate and depth of breathing).
- The patient's inspiratory-to-expiratory ratio (I:E ratio).
- Retractions of the intercostal spaces during inspiration.
- Nasal flaring.
- Pursed lip breathing.
- Symmetry of the chest.
- Whether the scapulae are symmetric and the spine is straight.
- Whether the excursion of the chest wall is symmetric. Does the diaphragm move downward and the thoracic cage move upward and outward during each inspiration?
- Whether the patient is splinting in an attempt to control chest pain by decreasing chest excursion. Splinting suggests the presence of pneumonia, rib fractures, pleural effusion, pneumothorax, or postoperative pain.
- The presence or absence of paradoxical movement of the lower costal margins. During the advanced stages of chronic obstructive pulmonary disease the costal margins first expand on inspiration and then contract.
- The patient's skin condition and color. Does the patient appear dehydrated? Does the skin appear cyanotic?

- Whether the patient's hands and nail beds manifest cyanosis and digital clubbing.
- The type of cough produced by the patient.
- The presence of audible wheezing or rhonchi.
- Whether there is evidence of distended neck and face veins and edema of the extremities—indications of congestive heart failure.
- Surgical scars.
- The presence of a "barrel chest."

External Landmarks

In an examination of the chest and lungs, various anatomic landmarks and imaginary vertical lines drawn on the chest are useful in pinpointing abnormal findings.

Anteriorly, the first rib and its cartilage are fastened to the manubrium directly beneath the clavicle. The second rib and its cartilage are adjacent to the sternal angle. The ribs can be easily numbered once the second rib is identified. The seventh rib and its cartilage are located on the sternum just above the xiphoid process. Anteriorly, the lungs normally extend to about the level of the xiphoid process (Fig 1–2).

Posteriorly, the ribs can be numbered by identifying the inferior angle of the scapulae. The seventh and eighth ribs lie near this point. The examiner may also trace the location of a rib from the front of the chest to the back. In the back the lungs normally extend to the level of the ninth or tenth rib (see Fig 1–2).

As shown in Figure 1–3 a good method for localizing certain findings is to use a reference grid of the following imaginary vertical lines drawn on the chest:

- Midsternal line
- Midclavicular line
- Anterior axillary line
- Midaxillary line
- Posterior axillary line
- Midscapular line
- Vertebral line

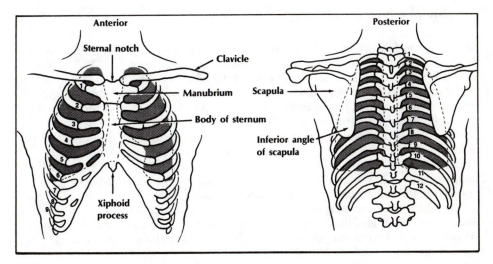

FIG 1–2.
Anatomic landmarks of the chest.

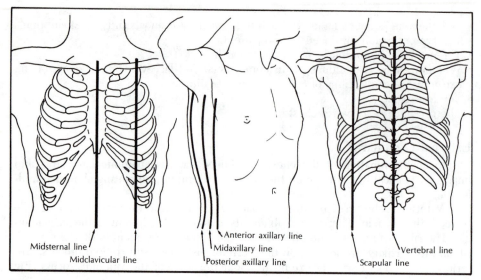

FIG 1–3.
Imaginary vertical lines of the chest.

Palpation

Palpation is the process of touching the patient in an effort to evaluate (1) areas of tenderness, (2) tone of the respiratory muscles, (3) any chest abnormalities that are not evident, and (4) fremitus.

When palpating the patient's chest for tenderness, muscle tone, and abnormalities, the examiner may use the heel of the hand, the ulnar surface of the hand, or the fingertips. The position of the patient's trachea, for example, can be determined by placing the index finger into the sternal notch.

Tactile and Vocal Fremitus

Vibration felt over the chest—produced by gas flowing through partially obstructed tracheobronchial segments—is known as tactile fremitus. The vibration caused by phonation and transmitted through the chest is called vocal fremitus. Vocal fremitus is commonly produced by the patient repeating the number "ninety-nine." Palpation should be performed from the top of the chest down and should be done both anteriorly and posteriorly (Fig 1–4).

Decreased tactile and vocal fremitus is caused by respiratory disorders that interfere with the transmission of sounds. Such respiratory problems include (1) chronic obstructive pulmonary disease accompanied by an elevated functional residual capacity, (2) tumors of the pleural cavity, and (3) pleural effusion.

When the pulmonary disorder produces consolidation within the lungs, tactile and vocal fremitus increase because liquid and solid materials transmit vibrations more readily than air-filled spaces do. Some causes of increased vocal fremitus are (1) pneumonia, (2) alveolar collapse or atelectasis, (3) pulmonary edema, (4) lung masses, and (5) pulmonary fibrosis.

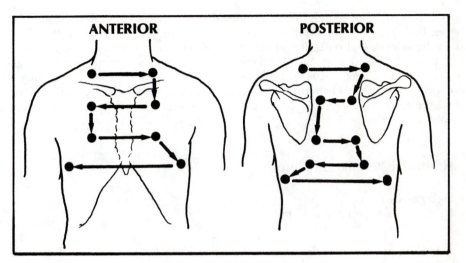

FIG 1–4.
Path of vocal or tactile fremitus.

Percussion

Percussion of the chest wall is performed to obtain information concerning the presence of air or consolidation within the chest cavity. When percussing the chest, the examiner firmly presses the distal portion of the middle finger of the nondominant hand onto the surface to be examined. No other part of the hand should touch the patient. Using the tip of the middle finger of the dominant hand, the examiner quickly strikes the distal joint of the positioned finger and then immediately withdraws the tapping finger (Fig 1–5). The sounds produced by percussion are re-

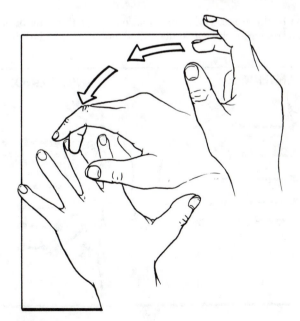

FIG 1–5.
Chest percussion technique.

different sampling proportions, however, you must learn or seek professional help to create a differential weighting scheme to adjust for the distortion of the results.

Sometimes you may want to employ some of the nonrandom sampling procedures discussed earlier with stratification. In such cases, the sample size for each category or stratum is not decided based on the power consideration but arbitrarily designated as a quota, and thus called quota sampling rather than stratified sampling. Stratified sampling is random while quota sampling is nonrandom. The two sampling procedures should not be confused with each other, although they are somewhat similar and both represent certain improvement of the sample representativeness.

Cluster sampling (sometimes called "area sampling"), on the other hand, is a very different sampling technique employing an opposite principle for stratification. This principle requires large (ideally, the maximum) differences within a cluster or area, but small (ideally, no) difference between clusters or areas. When similar heterogeneous groupings are available, one or a couple of them can be chosen to represent all the rest clusters or areas. In such cases, every unit in the selected cluster(s) will be studied and the cases or units as a whole will represent the entire research population. The sampling error depends on the differences between the clusters, and the random sampling of the clusters is crucial to the representativeness of the total sample. All the random sampling procedures discussed above may be used to select the clusters, though sampling clusters tend to be cheaper but less effective in controlling errors. Since this is the only technique that does not require you to list all the individual cases in the research population, you may not even know your sample size beforehand if the clusters are unequal-sized. Fortunately, people seldom use the cluster sampling technique alone. It is only used at one or a few stages in a multistage sampling process, in which you can predetermine your final sample size by applying additional procedures to sample individual cases or units.

Multistage sampling is a way for ambitious researchers to draw conclusion about the full range of a huge population without being able to list all the elements. This is done by using cluster sampling, i.e., the sampling of some listable groups of cases, units, or elements, at the initial stages, and then listing and selecting the individual cases (subjects) within each group or cluster by some of the basic random sampling procedures. To be able to infer the findings of the sample study on a very limited number of cases to the entire research population through such a procedure, you must ensure that the selection at each stage is

ferred to as resonant sounds. The examiner should percuss from the top down, between the ribs, and compare the sounds generated on the two sides of the chest. Both the anterior and posterior aspects of the chest should be percussed (Fig 1–6).

In a normal lung unit, the sound created by percussion is transmitted throughout the air-filled lung and is typically described as loud, low in pitch, and long in duration. The sounds elicited by the examiner vibrate freely throughout the large surface area of the lungs and create a sound like that elicited by knocking on an empty barrel (Fig 1–7).

Abnormal Percussion Notes

• Dull percussion note
• Hyperresonant percussion note

In persons with chest disorders such as pleural thickening, pleural effusion, atelectasis, or consolidation, the sound elicited on percussion does not resonate throughout the lungs. The sounds produced are typically described as dull, or soft, high in pitch, short in duration, and suggestive of those produced by knocking on a full barrel (Fig 1–8).

When the chest is percussed over areas of trapped gas, a hyperresonant note is produced. These sounds are typically described as very loud, low in pitch, long in duration, and reminiscent of those produced by knocking on an empty barrel (Fig 1–9). Such sounds are commonly elicited in patients with chronic obstructive pulmonary disease and in patients with pneumothorax.

Auscultation

Auscultation of the lungs yields information about the flow of gas through the tracheobronchial tree and the presence of alveolar consolidation, secretions, or

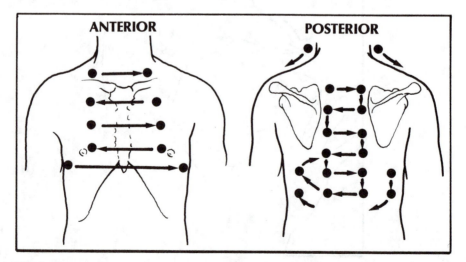

FIG 1–6.
Path of percussion.

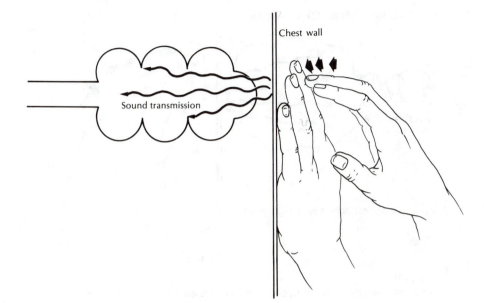

FIG 1–7.
Chest percussion of a normal lung.

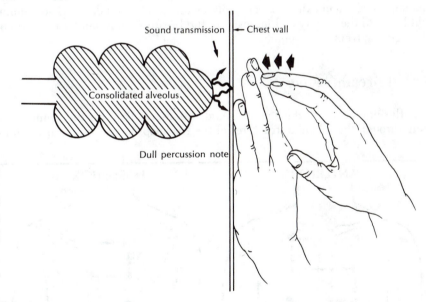

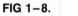

FIG 1–8.
A short, dull percussion note is typically produced over areas of alveolar consolidation.

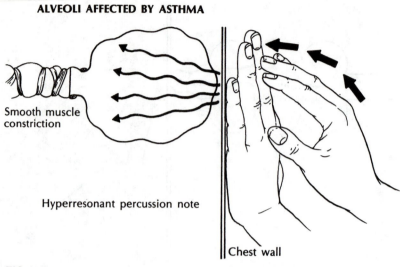

FIG 1–9.
Percussion becomes more hyperresonant with alveolar hyperinflation.

bronchial obstruction. The examiner should auscultate the chest from one side to the other and from top to bottom (Fig 1–10). Each area should be listened to while the patient inhales and exhales at a slightly increased rate and depth. The examiner should listen to the quality and intensity of the breath sounds and for the presence or absence of adventitious sounds.

Normal Breath Sounds

In the normal lung, the sounds heard on auscultation are the sounds of air rushing through the tubelike structures of the tracheobronchial tree. Since the rate

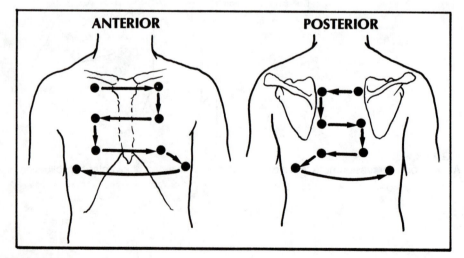

FIG 1–10.
Path of auscultation.

of flow changes very markedly between the trachea and the alveoli, the nature and pitch of the breath sounds change also.

Over the trachea and larger bronchi, the sound is loud and high-pitched and has a so-called tubular or bronchial quality. Such sounds are commonly referred to as normal bronchial breath sounds. Bronchial breath sounds may be louder during expiration, and there is generally a pause between the inspiratory phase and the expiratory phase.

Over the parenchymal areas of normal lungs, the breath sounds are much softer, have a lower pitch, and are much more evident during inspiration. This softer, lower-pitched sound over the parenchymal areas is due largely to the fact that the gas molecules entering the alveoli spread out over a larger surface area and therefore create less gas turbulence. As gas turbulence decreases, breath sounds decrease. The sounds are referred to as *bronchovesicular* or *vesicular sounds* (Fig 1–11).

Abnormal Breath Sounds

- Bronchial breath sounds
- Diminished breath sounds
- Crackles and rhonchi
- Wheezing
- Pleural friction rub
- Whispered pectoriloquy

Bronchial Breath Sounds.—If gas molecules are not permitted to dissipate throughout the parenchymal area (because of alveolar consolidation or atelectasis, for example) the gas molecules have no opportunity to spread out over a larger surface area and therefore become less turbulent. Consequently, the sounds produced in this area will be louder since the gas sounds are coming mainly from the tracheobronchial tree and not the lung parenchyma. These sounds are called *bronchial sounds.*

When students first think about bronchial breath sounds caused by alveolar consolidation or collapse, it is commonly argued that the breath sounds should be

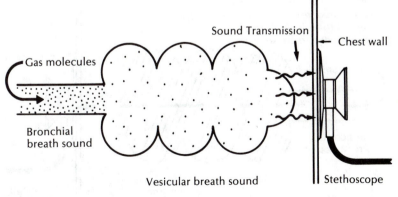

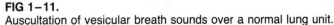

FIG 1–11.
Auscultation of vesicular breath sounds over a normal lung unit.

diminished since the consolidation acts as a sound barrier. While it may be true that alveolar collapse or consolidation does act as a sound barrier and so reduces bronchial breath sounds, the reduction is not as great as it would be if the gas molecules were allowed to dissipate throughout the lung parenchyma. In addition, liquid and solid materials transmit sounds more readily than air-filled spaces do and therefore may further contribute to the bronchial quality of the breath sound. Thus, when disease causes alveolar collapse or consolidation, there will be harsher, bronchial-type sounds over the affected areas rather than the normal vesicular sounds (Fig 1–12).

Diminished Breath Sounds.—Breath sounds are commonly diminished or distant when auscultated in respiratory disorders that lead to hypoventilation, regardless of the cause. For example, patients with chronic obstructive pulmonary disease commonly have diminished breath sounds. These patients hypoventilate because of the air trapping and increased functional residual capacity associated with obstructive lung disease. In addition, when the functional residual capacity is elevated, the gas that does enter the enlarged alveoli during each breath spreads out over a greater-than-normal surface area, thereby resulting in less gas turbulence and a softer sound (Fig 1–13). Heart sounds may also be diminished in patients with elevated functional residual capacity.

Diminished breath sounds are also found in respiratory disorders that cause hypoventilation by compressing the lung. Such disorders include flail chest, pleural effusion, and pneumothorax. Diminished breath sounds are also characteristic of neuromuscular diseases that cause hypoventilation. Such disorders include the Guillain-Barré syndrome and myasthenia gravis.

Crackles and Rhonchi.—Adjectives used in the older literature to describe crackles and rhonchi (moist, wet, dry, crackling, sibilant, coarse, fine, crepitant) depend largely on the auditory acuity and experience of the examiner. They have little value because it is only the presence or absence of crackles or rhonchi that is important. When fluid accumulation is present in a respiratory disorder, there are almost always some crackles or rhonchi, i.e., "bubbly" or "slurpy" sounds accompanying the breath sounds.

Crackles (formerly called rales) are usually fine or medium crackling wet sounds and are typically heard during inspiration. Crackles are formed in the small and medium-sized airways and generally do not change in nature after a strong, vigorous cough.

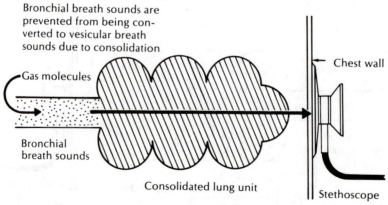

Bronchial breath sounds are prevented from being converted to vesicular breath sounds due to consolidation

Gas molecules

Chest wall

Bronchial breath sounds

Consolidated lung unit

Stethoscope

FIG 1–12.
Auscultation of bronchial breath sounds over a consolidated lung unit.

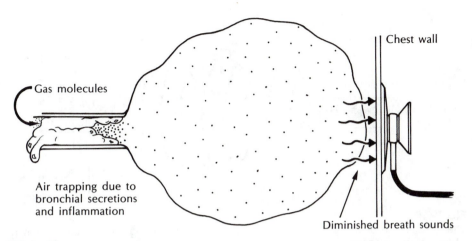

FIG 1–13.
As air trapping and alveolar hyperinflation develop in obstructive lung diseases, breath sounds progressively diminish.

Rhonchi, on the other hand, usually have a coarse, "bubbly" quality and are typically heard during expiration. Rhonchi are formed in the larger airways and often change in nature or cannot be heard after a strong, vigorous cough.

Wheezing.—Wheezing is the characteristic sound produced by bronchospasm. It is found in all bronchospastic disorders and is one of the cardinal findings in bronchial asthma. The sounds are high-pitched and whistling and generally last throughout the expiratory phase. The mechanism of a wheeze is similar to a vibrating reed of a woodwind instrument. The reed, which partially occludes the mouthpiece of the instrument, vibrates and produces a sound when air is forced through it (Fig 1–14).

Pleural Friction Rub.—If pleuritis accompanies a respiratory disorder, the inflamed pleural membranes resist movement during breathing and create a peculiar and very characteristic sound known as a pleural friction rub. The sound is reminis-

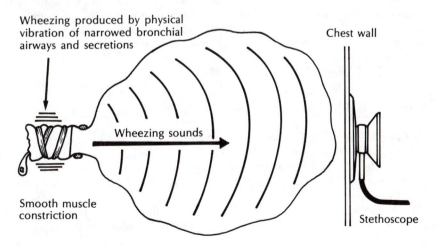

FIG 1–14.
Wheezing and rhonchi often develop during an asthmatic episode because of smooth muscle constriction and mucus production.

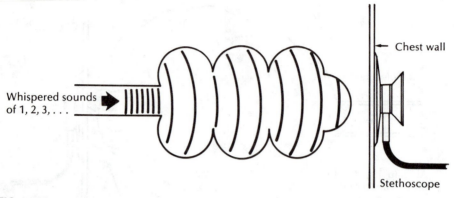

FIG 1–15.
The auscultation of whispered voice sounds over a normal lung unit are usually diminished and unintelligible.

cent of the sound made by a creaking shoe and is usually heard in the area where the patient complains about pain.

Whispered Pectoriloquy.—*Whispered pectoriloquy* is the term used to describe the unusually clear transmission of the whispered voice of a patient as heard through the stethoscope.

When the patient whispers a phrase like "one, two, three," the sounds produced by the vocal cords are transmitted not only toward the mouth and nose but throughout the lungs as well. As the whispered sounds travel down the tracheobronchial tree, they remain relatively unchanged, but as the sound disperses throughout the large surface areas of the alveoli, it diminishes sharply. Consequently, when one listens with a stethoscope over a normal lung unit while a patient whispers the phrase "one, two, three," the sounds are diminished, distant, and unintelligible (Fig 1–15).

When a patient who has atelectasis or consolidated lung areas whispers "one, two, three," the sounds produced are prevented from spreading out over a large alveolar surface area. Even though the consolidated area may act as a sound barrier and diminishes the sounds somewhat, the reduction in sounds is not as great as if the sounds were allowed to dissipate throughout a normal lung. Consequently, the whispered sounds will seem much louder and more intelligible over the affected lung areas (Fig 1–16).

Review of Normal Heart Sounds

Although there is still disagreement as to their exact origin, it is generally accepted that heart sounds develop in response to sudden changes in blood flow inside the heart that cause the walls of the heart chamber, the valves, and the great vessels to vibrate. It is the vibration of these heart-related structures that produces the heart sounds.

When the valves of the heart close, a "lubb-dub" sound is produced. The "lubb" sound is the first heart sound, or S_1. The "dub" sound is the second heart sound, or S_2.

S_1 is associated with the closure of the atrioventricular (AV) valves, i.e., the mitral and tricuspid valves (Fig 1–17). Both the mitral and the tricuspid valves pro-

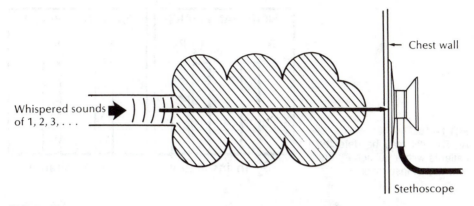

FIG 1–16.
The auscultation of whispered voice sounds over a consolidated lung unit are usually louder and more intelligible in comparison to a normal lung unit.

duce separate sounds within S_1; these are referred to as M_1 and T_1. S_1 corresponds to the onset of systole and is louder, longer, and lower pitched than S_2 at the apex. Closure of the mitral valve precedes closure of the tricuspid valve by 0.02 to 0.03 seconds as the ventricles begin to contract. Because the left ventricle is larger and more powerful than the right, however, the mitral valve closes with greater force than the tricuspid valve does and therefore is the major source of S_1 under normal circumstances.

S_2 results from closure of the semilunar valves, i.e., the aortic and pulmonic valves. The aortic and pulmonic valves each generate a separate sound within S_2; these are referred to as A_2 and P_2 (see Fig 1–17). An S_2 split of 0.03 to 0.07 seconds may be detected under normal circumstances by a trained examiner. Such a split, however, is noted only during inspiration (Fig 1–18).

The mechanism responsible for the S_2 split is as follows: during inspiration intrapleural pressure decreases, which causes venous blood to rush into the thorax. This action increases right ventricular stroke volume, which in turn delays pulmonary valve closure. At the same time, the increase in negative intrapleural pressure causes blood vessels in the lungs to dilate and retain blood. This action reduces left ventricular stroke volume and left ventricular systole. As a result, the aortic valve closes earlier. Finally, even though the closure of the aortic valve still precedes closure of the pulmonic valve during expiration, the closure sequence is so rapid that A_2 and P_2 are generally heard as a single sound.

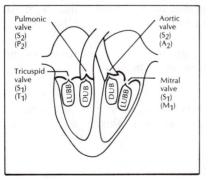

FIG 1–17.
Origin of the lubb-dub sound of the heart.

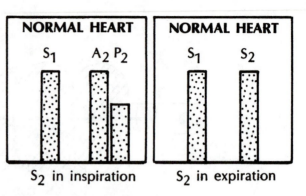

FIG 1–18.
An S_2 split may be detected i patients with a pulmonary embolism during inspiration.

OTHER COMMON CLINICAL MANIFESTATIONS

Cyanosis

Cyanosis is often seen in severe respiratory disorders. *Cyanosis* is the term used to describe the blue-gray or purplish discoloration seen on the mucous membranes, fingertips, and toes whenever the blood in these areas contains at least 5 gm/dL of reduced hemoglobin. When the normal 14 to 15 gm/dL of hemoglobin is fully saturated, the Pa_{O_2} will be about 97 to 100 mm Hg, and there will be about 20 vol% of oxygen in the blood. In a cyanotic patient with one third (5 gm/dL) of the hemoglobin reduced, the Pa_{O_2} will be about 30 mm Hg and there will be 13 vol% of oxygen in the blood (Fig 1–19).

The detection and interpretation of cyanosis is difficult, and there is wide individual variation between observers. The recognition of cyanosis depends on the acuity of the observer, on the light conditions in the examining room, and on the pigmentation of the patient. Cyanosis of the nail beds is also influenced by the temperature since vasoconstriction induced by cold may slow circulation to the point where the blood becomes bluish in the surface capillaries even though the arterial blood in the major vessels is not oxygen poor.

Central cyanosis, as observed on the mucous membranes of the mouth, is almost always a sign of hypoxemia and so has a definite diagnostic and prognostic value.

In the severely anemic patient, cyanosis may never be seen since these patients could not remain alive with 5 gm/dL reduced hemoglobin. In the patient with *polycythemia*,* however, cyanosis may be present at a Pa_{O_2} well above 30 mm Hg since the amount of reduced hemoglobin is often greater than 5 gm/dL in these patients—even when their total oxygen transport is within normal limits.

In respiratory disease, cyanosis is the end result of (1) a decreased ventilation-perfusion ratio, (2) pulmonary shunting, and (3) venous admixture.

Ventilation-Perfusion

Ideally, each alveolus in the lungs should receive the same ratio of ventilation and pulmonary capillary blood flow. In reality, however, this is not the case.

*See the section on polycythemia, page 67.

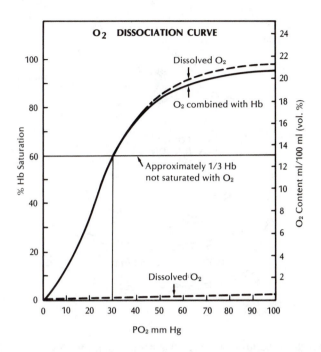

FIG 1–19.
Cyanosis is likely whenever the blood contains at least 5 gm of reduced hemoglobin. In the normal individual who has about 15 gm of hemoglobin per 100 mL of blood, a Po_2 of about 30 mm Hg will produce 5 gm of reduced hemoglobin. The hemoglobin, however, is still approximately 60% saturated with oxygen.

Alveolar ventilation is normally about 4 L/min and the pulmonary capillary blood flow is about 5 L/min, which makes the ratio of ventilation to blood flow 4:5, or 0.8. This relationship is referred to as the *ventilation-perfusion ($\dot{V}/\dot{Q}$) ratio* (Fig 1–20).

In a normal individual in the upright position, the alveoli in the upper portions of the lungs (apices) receive moderate amounts of ventilation and little blood flow. Consequently, the $\dot{V}/\dot{Q}$ ratio throughout this region is higher than 0.8. In the lower regions of the lung, alveolar ventilation is moderately increased, and the blood flow is greatly increased since blood flow is *gravity dependent*. As a result, the $\dot{V}/\dot{Q}$ ratio is lower than 0.8 in this area. In short, the $\dot{V}/\dot{Q}$ ratio progressively decreases from the top to the bottom of the lungs in an individual in the upright position, and the overall average $\dot{V}/\dot{Q}$ ratio is about 0.8. In respiratory disorders, the $\dot{V}/\dot{Q}$ ratio is usually altered.

Increased Ventilation-Perfusion Ratio.—In some disorders such as right-heart failure, the lungs receive little or no blood flow in relation to ventilation. When this condition develops, the $\dot{V}/\dot{Q}$ ratio increases. As a result, a larger portion of the alveolar ventilation will not be physiologically effective and is said to be "wasted" or "*dead-space*" *ventilation* (Fig 1–21). Generally, when the $\dot{V}/\dot{Q}$ ratio increases, the Pa_{O_2} increases and the Pa_{CO_2} decreases.

Decreased Ventilation-Perfusion Ratio.—In other lung disorders such as asthma or pneumonia, the lungs receive little or no ventilation in relation to blood flow. When this condition develops, the $\dot{V}/\dot{Q}$ ratio decreases. As a result, a larger portion

random, and be aware that the sampling error will be amplified by the number of stages involved. Unfortunately, in selecting some large clusters such as cities or counties, people tend to use procedures other than random selection, such as purposive or quota sampling. It is not justified to draw conclusions about the intended research population based on such sample studies. More prudent researchers would rather limit their definition of the research population to what is actually covered in the selected clusters or areas.

To recapitulate, major steps in sampling include: (1) defining the analytic unit (a "case") and the population; (2) deciding on sampling methods; (3) determining the sample size (based on the key variables) and sampling fractions; (4) establishing sampling frames (lists); (5) selecting cases; and (6) assessing sampling errors (e.g., missing patterns).

Longitudinal study and experimental design

Many research projects do not pursue the time dimension. In other words, they are not concerned with the change of the subjects and objects over time. Rather, they even try to avoid the influence of such change. Although those projects may ask questions about the past as well as the future, they themselves are not designed to follow through the process of change. They are done at one time and only examine a dissection or cross section in the time sequence. Since the time sequence of the changing states is critical in determining causation, cross-sectional studies are often conducted only at the exploratory or the descriptive level. Although people have reasons to argue for the explaining power of cross-sectional investigations, empirical researchers tend to adopt a longitudinal design if their aim is to draw some cause-effect conclusions. Nevertheless, as we will see soon, longitudinal studies also face some fatal problems that may keep them from drawing accurate cause-effect conclusions.

A longitudinal design of research is usually more complicated and costly than a cross-sectional study. By saying this, it is not meant that cross-sectional research will necessarily be simple and easy. For example, it could be very hard just to make it really cross-sectional since it is usually impossible to get an investigation done exactly at one point in time. It is not uncommon for a large-scale survey to take several weeks or even months to complete. Obviously, if it lasts that long the value of the project as cross-sectional research may depreciate rapidly and substantially, which may cause tremendous problems in data

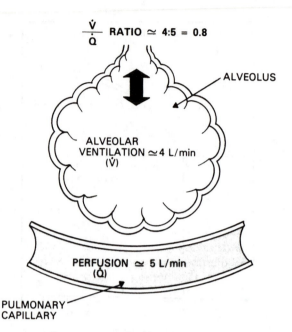

$$\frac{\dot{V}}{\dot{Q}} \text{ RATIO} \simeq 4{:}5 = 0.8$$

ALVEOLUS

ALVEOLAR
VENTILATION ≃ 4 L/min
(V̇)

PERFUSION ≃ 5 L/min
(Q̇)

PULMONARY
CAPILLARY

FIG 1–20.
The normal ventilation-perfusion ratio *(V̇/Q̇)* is about 0.8. (From Des Jardins TR: *Cardiopulmonary Anatomy and Physiology: Essentials for Respiratory Care.* Albany, NY, Delmar Publishers Inc, 1988. Used by permission.)

of the pulmonary blood flow will not be physiologically effective in terms of molecular gas exchange and is said to be "shunted" blood (see the section on pulmonary shunting below). Generally, when the V̇/Q̇ ratio decreases, the Pa_{O_2} decreases, and the Pa_{CO_2} increases.

Pulmonary Shunting

There are three forms of pulmonary shunting: the anatomic shunt, the capillary shunt, and the shuntlike effect.

Anatomic Shunt.—An anatomic shunt exists when blood flows from the right side of the heart to the left side without going through the pulmonary capillaries (Fig 1–22,B). Normally, this is about 2% to 5% of the cardiac output. This normal shunted blood comes from the bronchial, pleural, and thebesian veins. Such shunting can also be caused by congenital heart diseases, intrapulmonary fistulas, and pulmonary vascular abnormalities.

Capillary Shunt.—A capillary shunt is commonly caused by (1) alveolar collapse or atelectasis, (2) alveolar fluid accumulation, and (3) alveolar consolidation (see Fig 1–22,C). The sum of the anatomic and capillary shunts is referred to as a true or absolute shunt. Patients with respiratory disorders causing capillary shunting conditions will be refractory to oxygen therapy since the alveoli are unable to accommodate any form of ventilation.

Shuntlike Effect.—When pulmonary capillary perfusion is in excess of alveolar ventilation, a shuntlike effect can develop. Common causes of this form of shunting are (1) hypoventilation, (2) uneven distribution of ventilation (e.g., bronchospasm or excessive mucus accumulation in the tracheobronchial tree), and (3) alveolar-capillary diffusion defects (even though the alveolus may be ventilated in this condition, the

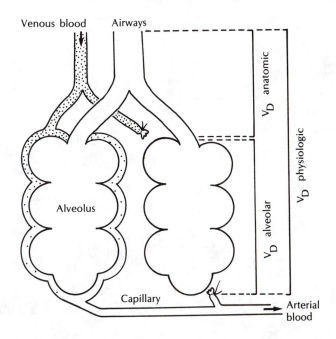

FIG 1–21.
Dead-space ventilation (VD).

Only the inspired air that reaches the alveoli is physiologically effective. This portion of the inspired gas is referred to as alveolar ventilation. The volume of inspired air that does not reach the alveoli is not physiologically effective. This portion of gas is referred to as dead-space ventilation. There are three types of deadspaces: anatomic, alveolar, and physiologic.

Anatomic dead space. Anatomic dead space refers to the volume of gas in the conducting airways: the nose, mouth, pharynx, larynx, and lower portions of the airways down to but not including the respiratory bronchioles. The volume of the anatomic dead space is approximately equal to 1 mL/lb. (2.2 mL/kg) of normal body weight.

Alveolar dead space. When an alveolus is ventilated but not perfused with blood, the volume of air in the alveolus is dead space, that is, the air within the alveolus is not physiologically effective in terms of gas exchange. The amount of alveolar dead space is unpredictable.

Physiologic dead space. The physiologic dead space is the sum of the anatomic dead space and the alveolar dead space. Since neither of these two forms of dead space is physiologically effective in terms of gas exchange, the two forms are combined and are referred to as physiologic dead space. (See Physiologic Deadspace Calculation, Appendix XIV.)

blood passing by the alveolus does not have time to equilibrate with the alveolar oxygen tension) (see Fig 1–22,C). Pulmonary shunting due to these conditions can generally be corrected by oxygen therapy.

Table 1–2 list some respiratory disorders associated with capillary shunting and shuntlike effects.

Venous Admixture

The end result of pulmonary shunting is venous admixture, which is the mixing of shunted, nonreoxygenated blood with reoxygenated blood distal to the alveoli (i.e., downstream in the pulmonary venous system) (Fig 1–23). When venous admixture occurs, the shunted, nonreoxygenated blood gains oxygen molecules while,

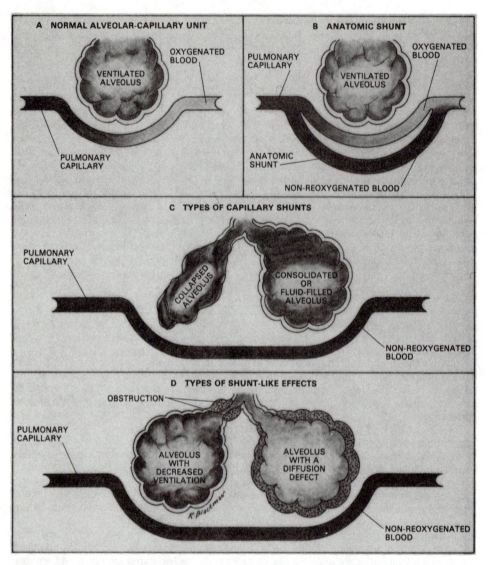

FIG 1–22.
Pulmonary shunting. *A* = normal alveolar-capillary unit; *B* = anatomic shunt; *C* = types of capillary shunts; *D* = types of shuntlike effects. (From Des Jardins TR: *Cardiopulmonary Anatomy and Physiology: Essentials for Respiratory Care.* Albany, NY, Delmar Publishers Inc, 1988. Used by permission.)

at the same time, the reoxygenated blood loses oxygen molecules. The reason for this is as follows:

1. The high Po_2 of the reoxygenated blood acts according to Henry's law, that is, oxygen molecules within the reoxygenated blood (high Po_2) quickly move into or expand throughout the plasma of the nonreoxygenated blood (low Po_2). This causes the plasma Po_2 of the nonreoxygenated blood to increase and the plasma Po_2 of the reoxygenated blood to decrease.

2. These physiologic processes continue until (1) the entire plasma Po_2 is in equilibrium and (2) all the hemoglobin molecules carry an equal number of oxygen molecules.

TABLE 1–2.
Type of Pulmonary Shunting Associated With Common Respiratory Diseases

Respiratory Disease	Capillary Shunt	Shuntlike Effect
Chronic bronchitis		X
Emphysema		X
Asthma		X
Croup/epiglottitis		X
Bronchiectasis	X	X
Cystic fibrosis	X	X
Pneumoconiosis	X	X
Pneumonia	X	
Pulmonary edema	X	
Adult respiratory distress syndrome	X	
Flail chest	X	
Pneumothorax	X	
Pleural diseases	X	
Kyphoscoliosis	X	
Tuberculosis	X	
Fungal diseases	X	
Idiopathic (infant) respiratory distress syndrome	X	

3. The end result will be a blood mixture that has higher P_{O_2} and Ca_{O_2} values than in venous blood but lower Pa_{O_2} and Ca_{O_2} values than in the nonshunted arterial blood.

Clinically, it is this blood mixture that is evaluated downstream (e.g., from the radial artery) to assess the patient's arterial blood gases (see Table 1–5).

Shunt Equation

Since pulmonary shunting and venous admixture are common complications in respiratory disorders, knowledge of the degree of shunting is desirable in developing patient care plans. The amount of intrapulmonary shunting can be calculated by using the *classic shunt equation:*

$$\frac{\dot{Q}s}{\dot{Q}_T} = \frac{Cc_{O_2} - Ca_{O_2}}{Cc_{O_2} - C\bar{v}_{O_2}}$$

where $\dot{Q}s$ is the cardiac output that is shunted, $\dot{Q}_T$ is the total cardiac output, Cc_{O_2} is the oxygen content of capillary blood, Ca_{O_2} is the oxygen content of arterial blood, and $C\bar{v}_{O_2}$ is the oxygen content of venous blood.

In order to obtain the data necessary to calculate the patient's intrapulmonary shunting, the following clinical information must be gathered:

- Barometric pressure (PB)
- Pa_{O_2} (partial pressure of arterial oxygen)
- Pa_{CO_2} (partial pressure of arterial carbon dioxide)
- $P\bar{v}_{O_2}$ (partial pressure of mixed venous oxygen)
- Hemoglobin (Hb) concentration
- PA_{O_2} (partial pressure of alveolar oxygen)*
- FI_{O_2} (fractional concentration of inspired oxygen)

An example of the shunt calculation follows.

*See the ideal alveolar gas equation, Appendix XIII.

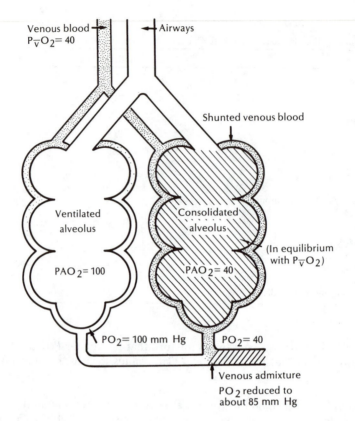

FIG 1–23.
Venous admixture occurs when reoxygenated blood mixes with non-reoxygenated blood distal to the alveoli.

Case Study: Automobile Accident Victim

A 22-year-old man is on a volume-cycled mechanical ventilator on a day when the barometric pressure is 755 mm Hg. The patient is receiving an FI_{O_2} of .60. The following clinical data are obtained:

- Hb: 15 gm/dL
- Pa_{O_2}: 65 mm Hg (Sa_{O_2} = 90%)
- Pa_{CO_2}: 56 mm Hg
- $P\bar{v}_{O_2}$ 35 mm Hg ($S\bar{v}_{O_2}$ = 65%)

With this information, the patient's Pa_{O_2}, Cc_{O_2}, Ca_{O_2}, and $C\bar{v}_{O_2}$ can now be calculated. (Remember that PH_2O represents alveolar water vapor pressure and is always considered 47 mm Hg.)

$$
\begin{aligned}
1.\ PA_{O_2} &= (PB - PH_2O)\, FI_{O_2} - Pa_{CO_2}\,(1.25) \\
&= (755 - 47)\,.60 - 56\,(1.25) \\
&= (708)\,.60 - 70 \\
&= (424.8) - 70 \\
&= 354.8
\end{aligned}
$$

2. Cc_{O_2} = (Hb × 1.34) + ($P_{A_{O_2}}$ × 0.003)
       = (15 × 1.34) + (354.8 × 0.003)
       = (20.1) + 1.064
       = 21.164 (vol% O_2)

3. Ca_{O_2} = (Hb × 1.34 × Sa_{O_2}) + (Pa_{O_2} × 0.003)
       = (15 × 1.34 × .90) + (65 × 0.003)
       = (18.09) + (0.195)
       = 18.285 (vol% O_2)

4. $C\bar{v}_{O_2}$ = (Hb × 1.34 × $S\bar{v}_{O_2}$) + ($P\bar{v}_{O_2}$ × 0.003)
       = (15 × 1.34 × .65) + (35 × 0.003)
       = (13.065) + (0.105)
       = 13.17 (vol% O_2)

With the results of these calculations, the patient's intrapulmonary shunting can now be calculated.

$$\frac{\dot{Q}s}{\dot{Q}T} = \frac{Cc_{O_2} - Ca_{O_2}}{Cc_{O_2} - C\bar{v}_{O_2}}$$

$$= \frac{21.164 - 18.285}{21.164 - 13.17}$$

$$= \frac{2.879}{7.994}$$

$$= 0.36$$

Thus, 36% of the patient's pulmonary blood flow is perfusing lung tissue that is not being ventilated.

With the proliferation of inexpensive personal computer systems, much of the shunt equation is now being written in simple programs. What was once a rather esoteric, error-prone procedure is now readily and accurately available to respiratory therapy practitioners.

Table 1–3 shows the clinical significance of pulmonary shunting.

Increased Respiratory Rate

On the basis of the anatomic alterations of the lung that are associated with the respiratory disorder, there may be several pathophysiologic mechanisms operating simultaneously that lead to an increased ventilatory rate. The major known mechanisms are as follows:

- Decreased lung compliance/increased work of breathing relationship
- Stimulation of central chemoreceptors
- Stimulation of the peripheral chemoreceptors
- Reflexes
  - Hering-Breuer inflation reflex
  - Deflation reflex
  - Irritant reflex
  - Juxtapulmonary-capillary receptors (J receptors)
  - Reflexes from the aortic and carotid sinus baroreceptors
- Pain/anxiety

TABLE 1–3.
Clinical Significance of Pulmonary Shunting

Degree of Pulmonary Shunting (%)	Clinical Significance
Below 10	Normal lung status
10–20	Indicates a pulmonary abnormality, but not significant in terms of cardiopulmonary support
20–30	May be life-threatening, and cardiopulmonary support may be needed
Greater than 30	Serious life-threatening condition, and cardiopulmonary support is almost always required

Decreased Lung Compliance/Increased Work of Breathing Relationship

How readily the elastic forces of the lungs accept a volume of inspired air is known as lung compliance (C_L). C_L is measured in terms of unit volume change per unit pressure change. Mathematically, it is written as liters per centimeter of water pressure. In other words, compliance determines how much air, in liters, the lungs will accommodate for each centimeter of water pressure change.

For example, when the normal individual generates a negative intrapleural pressure change of 2 cm H_2O during inspiration, the lungs accept a new volume of about 0.2 L gas. Thus, the C_L of the lungs would be expressed as 0.1 L/cm H_2O:

$$C_L = \frac{\Delta V \ (L)}{\Delta P \ (cm \ H_2O)}$$
$$= \frac{.2 \ L \ of \ gas}{2 \ cm \ H_2O}$$
$$= 0.1 \ L/cm \ H_2O \ (or \ 100 \ mL/cm \ H_2O)$$

The normal compliance of the lungs is graphically illustrated by the volume-pressure curve (Fig 1–24). When C_L increases, the lungs accept a greater volume of gas per unit pressure change. When C_L decreases, the lungs accept a smaller volume of gas per unit pressure change (Fig 1–25).

How Lung Compliance and Airway Resistance Affect Ventilatory Patterns.— An individual's ventilatory pattern is defined as (1) the rate at which the patient breathes per minute and (2) the tidal volume of each breath. Normally, the ventilatory rate is about 15 breaths per minute, and the tidal volume is about 500 mL. Although the precise mechanism is not clear, it is well documented that certain ventilatory patterns typically develop when lung compliance decreases and airway resistance increases.

When C_L decreases, the patient's breathing rate generally increases while, at the same time, the tidal volume decreases (Fig 1–26). This type of breathing pattern is commonly seen in restrictive lung disorders such as pneumonia, pulmonary edema, or adult respiratory distress syndrome. This breathing pattern is also com-

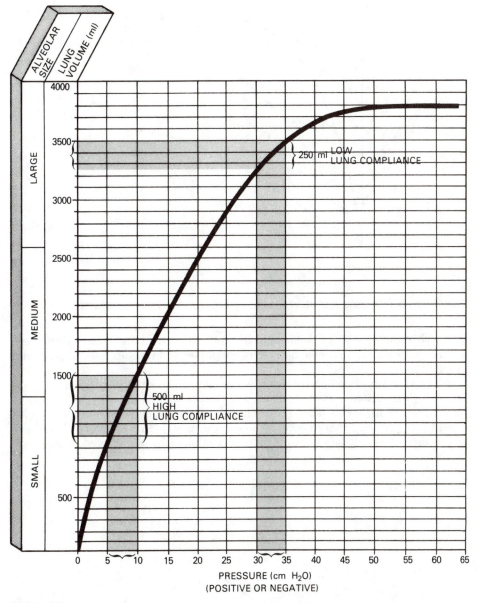

FIG 1–24.
Normal volume-pressure curve. The curve shows that lung compliance progressively decreases as the lungs get larger. For example, note the greater volume change between 5 and 10 cm H_2O (small/medium alveoli) than between 30 and 35 cm H_2O (large alveoli). (From Des Jardins TR: *Cardiopulmonary Anatomy and Physiology: Essentials for Respiratory Care.* Albany, NY, Delmar Publishers Inc, 1988. Used by permission.)

monly seen during the early stages of an acute asthmatic attack when the alveoli are hyperinflated—C_L progressively decreases as the alveolar volume increases (see Fig 1–24).

When airway resistance increases severely, the patient's breathing rate usually decreases while, at the same time, the tidal volume increases (see Fig 1–26). This

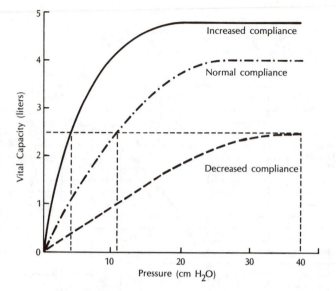

FIG 1–25.
The effects of increased and decreased compliance on the volume-pressure curve.

type of breathing pattern is commonly seen in obstructive lung diseases during the advanced stages (e.g., chronic bronchitis, emphysema, bronchiectasis, asthma, and cystic fibrosis).

The ventilatory pattern adopted by the patient in either a restrictive or obstructive lung disorder is thought to be based on minimum work requirements rather than ventilatory efficiency. In physics, work is defined as the force multiplied by the distance moved (work = force × distance). In respiratory physiology, the change in pulmonary pressure (force) multiplied by the change in lung vol-

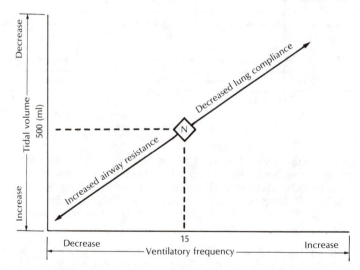

FIG 1–26.
The effects of increased airway resistance and decreased lung compliance on ventilatory frequency and tidal volume.

ume (distance) may be used to quantitate the amount of work required to breathe (work = pressure × volume).

It should be noted that the patient's adopted ventilatory pattern may not be seen in the clinical setting because of secondary heart or lung problems. For example, a patient with chronic emphysema who has adopted a decreased ventilatory rate and an increased tidal volume because of the increased airway resistance associated with the disorder will likely demonstrate an increased ventilatory rate and decreased tidal volume in response to a secondary lung infection (a restrictive lung disorder superimposed on a chronic obstructive lung disorder).

Thus, because the patient may adopt a ventilatory pattern based on the expenditure of energy rather than the efficiency of ventilation, it cannot be assumed that the ventilatory pattern acquired by the patient in response to a certain respiratory disorder is the most efficient one in terms of physiologic gas exchange.

Stimulation of Central Chemoreceptors

Although the mechanism is not fully understood, it is now believed that two special respiratory components in the medulla, called the dorsal respiratory group (DRG) and the ventral respiratory group (VRG), are responsible for coordinating respirations (Fig 1–27). Both the DRG and the VRG are stimulated by an excess concentration of hydrogen ions [H^+] in the cerebrospinal fluid (CSF). The H^+ concentration of the CSF is monitored by the central chemoreceptors, which are located bilaterally and ventrally in the substance of the medulla. A portion of the central chemoreceptors is actually in direct contact with the CSF. It is believed that

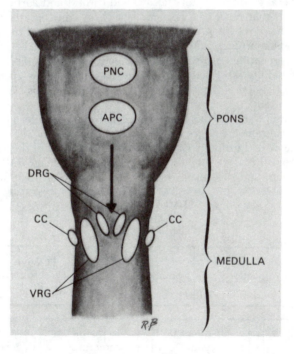

FIG 1–27.
Schematic illustration of the respiratory components of the lower brain stem (pons and medulla). *PNC* = pneumotaxic center; *APC* = apneustic center; *DRG* = dorsal respiratory group; *VRG* = ventral respiratory group; *CC* = central chemoreceptors. (From Des Jardins TR: *Cardiopulmonary Anatomy and Physiology: Essentials for Respiratory Care.* Albany, NY, Delmar Publishers Inc, 1988. Used by permission.)

analysis.

A longitudinal research, on the other hand, is designed to last a certain period of time, with the duration or the process being considered important or critical to the kind of questions to be answered. A longitudinal research, however, is not simply a prolonged cross-sectional study. It is more structured, and often composed of a series of cross-sectional data collection episodes, which form the basis of a most frequently seen type of analytic structure called time series analysis.

According to the characteristics of the research sample in a timed process, a longitudinal design may fall in one of the following three categories: panel study, cohort study, and trend study.

A panel design uses the same set of subjects, and studies them each time in a time series. This makes it possible to tell exactly what happened to the variables that constituted a case during the time period of change. Yet, a potential problem with this design is that it may be hard or impossible to retain all the cases in the research sample. Because the eligibility of people for the study is changing, and some are moving or even dying (especially when studying such special populations as the elderly and AIDS or cancer patients), it can be difficult to maintain the required sample size by continuing to study only the originally selected subjects. This problem is called panel attrition, and it may erode the representativeness of the original sample if some groups are more likely to drop out than others. Sometimes replacement sampling is held to provide additional subjects for study. Yet this alters the composition of the research sample and this will affect the ability of such design to render conclusive findings.

A cohort is an age group, or a group of people who were born or experienced some particular life events in a given period of time with certain eligibility for participation in the study. A cohort design does not use the same sample for the entire duration of study, but keeps sampling from the same population, i.e., people who were born or experienced the same thing in the same time period. Since the samples being studied are different from time to time, the change of the same people over time could be confused with the variation across different peoples. This approach does not have to face the problem of losing subjects, however. And choosing samples from the same population, i.e., people of the same experience (birth, marriage, and etc.) in the same year(s) would help rule out the variations caused simply by the shifting of the research population.

A trend study, in contrast, does not stick to the same population. Its definition of the research population allows for the turnover of its cases over time, or the

the central chemoreceptors transmit signals to the respiratory neurons by the following mechanism:

1. When the CO_2 level increases in the blood (e.g., during periods of hypoventilation), CO_2 molecules readily diffuse across the blood-brain barrier and enter the CSF. The blood-brain barrier is a semipermeable membrane that separates circulating blood from the CSF. The blood-brain barrier is relatively impermeable to ions like H^+ and HCO^-_3 but is very permeable to CO_2.

2. Once CO_2 crosses the blood-brain barrier and enters the CSF, it forms carbonic acid:

$$CO_2 + H_2O \leftrightarrows H_2CO_3 \leftrightarrows H^+ + HCO_3^-$$

3. Because the CSF has an inefficient buffering system, the H^+ produced from the above reaction rapidly increases and causes the pH level in the CSF to decrease.

4. The central chemoreceptors react to the liberated H^+ by sending signals to the respiratory components of the medulla, which in turn increase the ventilatory rate.

5. The increased ventilatory rate causes the Pa_{CO_2} and, subsequently, the P_{CO_2} in the CSF to decrease. Thus, the CO_2 level in the blood regulates ventilation by its indirect effect on the pH of the CSF (Fig 1–28).

Stimulation of the Peripheral Chemoreceptors

The peripheral chemoreceptors (also called carotid and aortic bodies) are oxygen-sensitive cells that react to a reduction of oxygen in the arterial blood (Pa_{O_2}). The peripheral chemoreceptors are located at the bifurcation of the internal and external carotid arteries (Fig 1–29) and on the aortic arch (Fig 1–30). Although the peripheral chemoreceptors are stimulated whenever the Pa_{O_2} is less than 500 mm Hg, they are generally most active when the Pa_{O_2} falls below 60 mm Hg (Sa_{O_2} of about 90%). Suppression of these chemoreceptors, however, is seen when the Pa_{O_2} falls below 30 mm Hg.

When the peripheral chemoreceptors are activated, an afferent (sensory) signal is sent to the respiratory centers of the medulla by way of the glossopharyngeal nerve (cranial nerve IX) from the carotid bodies and by way of the vagus nerve (cranial nerve X) from the aortic bodies. Efferent (motor) signals are then sent to the respiratory muscles, and this results in an increased rate of breathing.

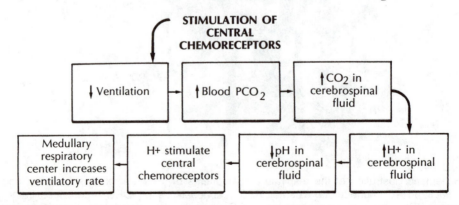

FIG 1–28.
The central chemoreceptors are stimulated by hydrogen ions *(H+)*, which increase in concentration as CO_2 moves into the CSF.

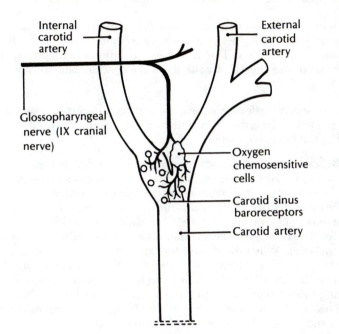

FIG 1–29.
Oxygen chemosensitive cells and the carotid sinus baroreceptors located on the carotid artery.

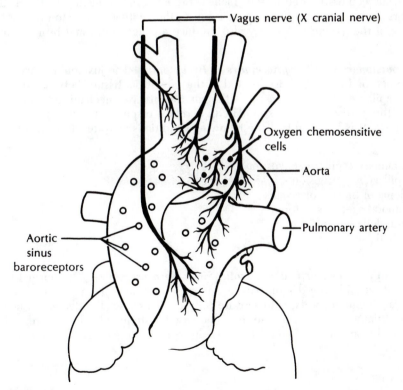

FIG 1–30.
Oxygen chemosensitive cells and the aortic sinus baroreceptors located on the aorta and pulmonary artery.

In patients who have a chronically low Pa_{O_2} and high Pa_{CO_2} (e.g., the advanced stages of emphysema), the peripheral chemoreceptors may be totally responsible for the control of ventilation. This is because a chronically high CO_2 concentration in the CSF inactivates the H^+ sensitivity of the central chemoreceptors.

Reflexes

There are several reflexes that may be activated in certain respiratory diseases, and these influence the patient's ventilatory rate. Some of the major reflexes are elaborated in the following sections.

Deflation Reflex.—When the lungs are compressed or deflated (e.g., atelectasis), an increased rate of breathing is seen. The precise mechanism responsible for this reflex is not known. Some investigators suggest that the increased rate of breathing may simply be due to reduced stimulation of the receptors serving the Hering-Breuer inflation reflex rather than the stimulation of specific deflation receptors. Receptors for the Hering-Breuer inflation reflex are located in the walls of the bronchi and bronchioles. When these receptors are stretched (e.g., during a deep inspiration), a reflex response is triggered to decrease the ventilatory rate. Others, however, feel that the deflation reflex is not due to the absence of receptor stimulation of the Hering-Breuer reflex since the reflex is still seen when the bronchi and bronchioles are below a temperature of 8° C. The Hering-Breuer reflex is not seen when the bronchi and bronchioles are below this temperature.

Irritant Reflex.—When the lungs are compressed, deflated, or exposed to noxious gases, the irritant receptors are stimulated. The irritant receptors are subepithelial mechanoreceptors located in the trachea, bronchi, and bronchioles. When the receptors are activated, a reflex response causes the ventilatory rate to increase. Stimulation of the irritant reflex may also produce a cough reflex and bronchoconstriction.

Juxtapulmonary-Capillary Receptors (J Receptors).—The juxtapulmonary-capillary receptors, or J receptors, are located in the interstitial tissues between the pulmonary capillaries and the alveoli. Although the precise mechanism is not known, when the J receptors are stimulated, a reflex response triggers rapid, shallow breathing. It is believed that the following conditions activate the J receptors:

- Pulmonary capillary congestion
- Capillary hypertension
- Edema of the alveolar walls
- Humoral agents (serotonin)
- Lung deflation
- Emboli

Reflexes From the Aortic and Carotid Sinus Baroreceptors.—The normal function of the aortic and carotid sinus baroreceptors, located near the aortic and carotid peripheral chemoreceptors, is to activate reflexes that cause (1) a decreased heart rate and ventilatory rate in response to an increased systemic blood pressure and (2) an increased heart rate and ventilatory rate in response to a decreased systemic blood pressure.

Pain/Anxiety

An increased respiratory rate may simply be due to the chest pain or fear and anxiety associated with the patient's inability to breath.

Pulmonary Function Findings in Restrictive and Obstructive Lung Disorders

Overview of Normal Lung Volumes and Capacities

As shown in Figure 1–31, air in the lungs is divided into four separate volumes. The four lung "capacities" represent different combinations of lung volumes.

Lung Volumes.—

- Tidal volume (V_T).—The volume of air that normally moves into and out of the lungs in one quiet breath.
- Inspiratory reserve volume (IRV).—The volume of air that can be forcefully inspired after a normal tidal volume inhalation.
- Expiratory reserve volume (ERV).—The volume of air that can be forcefully exhaled after a normal tidal volume exhalation.
- Residual volume (RV).—The amount of air remaining in the lungs after a forced exhalation.

Lung Capacities.—

- Vital capacity (VC).—VC = IRV + V_T + ERV. This is the volume of air that can be exhaled after a maximal inspiration. There are two major VC measurements: *slow vital capacity* (SVC), or a vital capacity in which exhalation is performed slowly, and *forced vital capacity* (FVC), or a vital capacity in which a maximal effort is made to exhale as rapidly as possible.
- Inspiratory capacity (IC).—IC = V_T + IRV. This is the volume of air that can be inhaled after a normal exhalation.

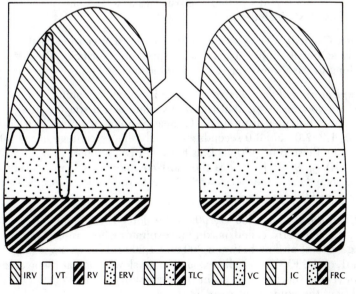

FIG 1–31.
Normal lung volumes and capacities. *IRV* = inspiratory reserve volume; V_T = tidal volume; *RV* = residual volume; *ERV* = expiratory reserve volume; *TLC* = total lung capacity; *VC* = vital capacity; *IC* = inspiratory capacity; *FRC* = functional residual capacity.

TABLE 1–4.

Lung Volumes and Capacities (in Milliliters) of Normal Recumbent Subject Between 20 and 30 Years of Age

Measurement	Male	Female
Tidal volume (V_T)	500	400–500
Inspiratory reserve volume (IRV)	3,100	1,900
Expiratory reserve volume (ERV)	1,200	800
Residual volume (RV)	1,200	1,000
Vital capacity (VC)	4,800	3,200
Inspiratory capacity (IC)	3,600	2,400
Functional residual capacity (FRC)	2,400	1,800
Total lung capacity (TLC)	6,000	4,200

- Functional residual capacity (FRC).— FRC = ERV + RV.
- Total lung capacity (TLC).— TLC = IC + FRC. This is the maximal amount of air that the lungs can accommodate.

The amount of air the lungs can accommodate varies with age, weight, height, and the sex of the individual. Table 1–4 lists the normal lung volumes and capacities of the average man and woman aged 20 to 30 years.

Overview of Expiratory Flow Rate Measurements

In addition to the volumes and capacities that can be measured by pulmonary function testing, it is also possible to measure the rate at which gas flows out of the lungs. Such measurements provide data on the integrity of the airways, the severity of airway impairment, and whether the patient has a large-airway or a small-airway problem. These tests include the following.

Forced Vital Capacity.— FVC is the volume of gas that can be exhaled as forcefully and rapidly as possible after a maximal inspiration. Normally FVC = VC. In obstructive lung disease, however, FVC is reduced (Fig 1–32).

Forced Expiratory Volume, Timed.— Forced expiratory volume, timed (FEV_T), is the maximum volume of gas that can be exhaled over a specific time period. This measurement is obtained from an FVC measurement. Commonly used time periods are 0.5, 1.0, 2.0, and 3.0 seconds. Normally the percentage of the total volume exhaled during these time periods is as follows: $FEV_{0.5}$, 60%; $FEV_{1.0}$, 83%; $FEV_{2.0}$, 94%; and $FEV_{3.0}$, 97%. $FEV_{1.0}$ is the most commonly used measurement. In obstructive disease, the time necessary to forcefully exhale a certain volume is increased (Fig 1–33).

Forced Expiratory Flow 200–1,200.— The forced expiratory flow 200–1,200, ($FEF_{200-1,200}$) (formerly called maximum expiratory flow rate [MEFR]) measures the average rate of airflow between 200 and 1,200 mL of an FVC (Fig 1–34). The first 200 mL of the FVC is usually exhaled more slowly than at the average flow rate because of (1) the inertia involved in the respiratory maneuver and (2) the general unreliability of the equipment response time.

Because the $FEF_{200-1,200}$ measures expiratory flows at high lung volumes (i.e., the initial part of the forced vital capacity), it is a good index of the integrity of large-airway function. The normal $FEF_{200-1,200}$ for the average healthy male be-

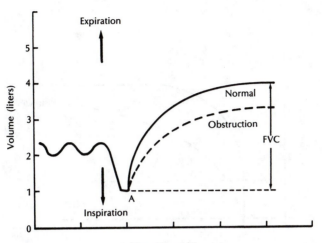

FIG 1–32.
Forced vital capacity *(FVC)*. *A* is the point of maximal inspiration and the starting point of an FVC.

tween 20 and 30 years of age is about 8 L/sec (480 L/min). The normal $FEF_{200-1,200}$ for the average healthy female between 20 and 30 years of age is about 5.5 L/sec (330 L/min). In obstructive lung disease, however, flow rates as low as 1 L/sec (60 L/min) have been reported. The $FEF_{200-1,200}$ is the most responsive test to bronchodilator therapy.

Forced Expiratory Flow 25%–75%.—The $FEF_{25\%-75\%}$ (also known as the maximum midexpiratory flow rate [MMFR]) is the average flow rate during the middle 50% of an FVC measurement (Fig 1–35). This expiratory maneuver is commonly used to assess the status of medium-sized airways in obstructive lung diseases. The normal $FEF_{25\%-75\%}$ for the average healthy male between 20 and 30 years of age

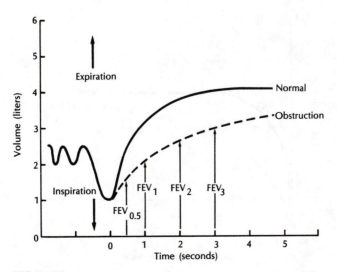

FIG 1–33.
Forced expiratory volume timed *(FEV$_T$)*.

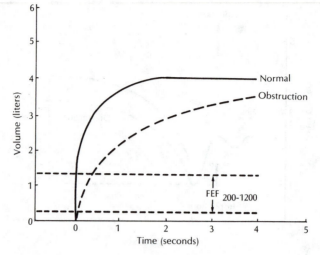

FIG 1–34.
Forced expiratory flow 200–1,200 *(FEF$_{200-1,200}$)*.

is about 4.5 L/sec (270 L/min). The normal FEF$_{25\%-75\%}$ for the average healthy female between 20 and 30 years of age is about 3.5 L/sec (210 L/min). The FEF$_{25\%-75\%}$ progressively decreases with age. In obstructive disease, flow rates as low as 0.3 L/sec (20 L/min) have been reported.

Peak Expiratory Flow Rate.—The peak expiratory flow rate (PEFR) (also known as the peak flow rate—[PF]) is the maximum flow rate that can be achieved. This measurement can be obtained from an FVC (Fig 1–36). The normal PEFR for the average healthy male between 20 and 30 years of age is about 10 L/sec (600 L/min). The normal PEFR for the average healthy female between 20 and 30 years of age is about 7.5 L/sec (450 L/min). The PEFR progressively decreases in obstructive disease.

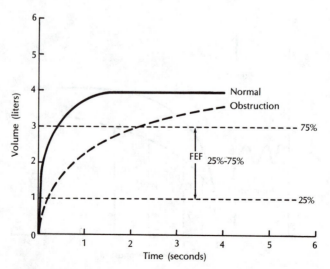

FIG 1–35.
Forced expiratory flow 25% to 75% *(FEF$_{25\%-75\%}$)*.

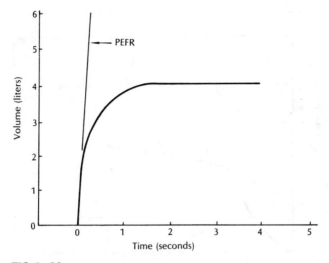

FIG 1–36.
Peak expiratory flow rate *(PEFR).*

Maximum Voluntary Ventilation.—The maximum voluntary ventilation (MVV) (also known as the maximum breathing capacity [MBC]) is the largest volume of gas that can be breathed voluntarily in and out of the lungs in 1 minute. The normal MVV for the average healthy male between 20 and 30 years of age is about 170 L/min. The normal MVV for the average healthy female between 20 and 30 years of age is about 110 L/min. The MVV progressively decreases in obstructive disease (Fig 1–37).

Forced Expiratory Volume in 1 Second/Forced Vital Capacity Ratio.—The FEV_1/ FVC ratio is also used as a broad indicator of airway obstruction. Although a decreased ratio is a reliable measurement of airway obstruction, the absence of a decreased ratio does not exclude the presence of airway obstruction.

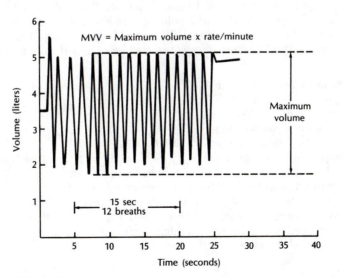

FIG 1–37.
Maximum voluntary ventilation *(MVV).*

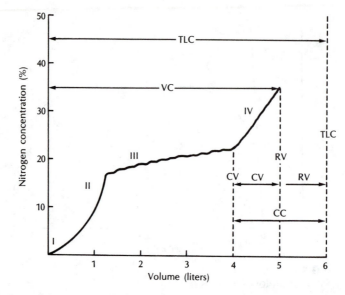

FIG 1–38.
Single-breath nitrogen test measurement for closing volume and capacity. *TLC* = total lung capacity; *VC* = vital capacity; *RV* = residual volume; *CC* = closing capacity.

Closing Volume and Closing Capacity.—Closing volume (CV) is the volume of gas, in excess of the residual volume (RV), that is trapped in the lungs as a result of small-airway closure during a normal (or slow) expiration. Closing capacity (CC) is the sum of the CV and RV and is written as a percentage of the total lung capacity.

Both of these pulmonary function findings are obtained from a single-breath nitrogen elimination (SBN_2) test. The results of an SBN_2 test are presented in four phases in Figure 1–38. The beginning of phase IV represents the onset of small-airway closure or air trapping.

Flow-Volume Loop.—As shown in Figure 1–39, the flow-volume loop illustrates a maximum forced expiration flow and volume (MEFV) curve, followed by a maximum inspiratory flow and volume (MIFV) curve. Depending on the sophistication of the equipment, the following information can be obtained from this test:

- Peak expiratory flow rate (PEFR)
- Peak inspiratory flow rate (PIFR)
- Forced vital capacity (FVC)
- Forced expiratory volume, timed (FEV_T)
- Forced expiratory flow, 25% to 75% ($FEF_{25\%-75\%}$)
- Forced expiratory flow, 50% ($FEF_{50\%}$).—This test is also called the $\dot{V}max_{50}$. In normal subjects, the $FEF_{50\%}$ has a straight-line appearance since the expiratory flow decreases linearly with volume throughout most of the vital capacity (VC) range. In subjects with obstructive lung disease, however, flow is frequently decreased at low lung volumes, and this causes the $FEF_{50\%}$ line to appear "cup-like" or "scooped out." There is a high correlation between the $FEF_{50\%}$ and $FEF_{25\%-75\%}$ in obstructive lung disease.

Flow-volume loop measurements graphically illustrate both obstructive lung problems (Fig 1–40) and restrictive lung problems (Fig 1–41).

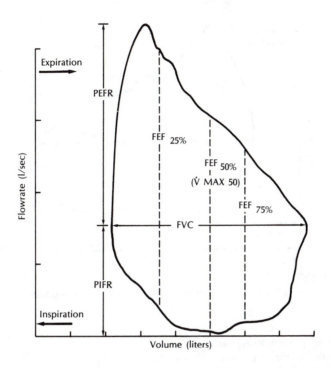

FIG 1–39.
Normal flow-volume loop. *PEFR* = peak expiratory flow rate; *PIFR* = peak inspiratory flow rate; *FVC* = forced vital capacity; *FEF$_{25\%-75\%}$* =. forced expiratory flow, 25% to 75%; *FEF$_{50\%}$* = forced expiratory flow 50% (also called Vmax$_{50}$).

Diffusion Capacity of Carbon Monoxide.—The diffusion capacity of the lung measures the amount of gas that moves across the alveolar-capillary membrane and into the blood. In essence, this test measures the physiologic effectiveness of the alveolar-capillary membrane. The normal diffusion capacity of carbon monoxide is 25 mL/min/mm Hg. The carbon monoxide single-breath technique is commonly used for this measurement.

Pulmonary Function Studies: Lung Volume and Capacity Findings Characteristic of a Restrictive Lung Disorder

- Decreased vital capacity (VC)
- Decreased residual volume (RV)
- Decreased functional residual capacity (FRC)
- Decreased total lung capacity (TLC)
- Decreased tidal volume (VT)

The above lung volumes and capacities develop in response to pathologic conditions that alter the anatomic structures distal to the terminal bronchials. Such conditions include the following:

- Lung compression (e.g., kyphoscoliosis or pleural effusion)
- Atelectasis (e.g., pneumothorax or flail chest)
- Consolidation (e.g., pneumonia)

Preface

Research is an integral part of higher education. It is especially important for those who are labeled as "research students" (usually honors and higher degree pursuers), faculty at so-called "research universities," and graduates working as researchers in various organizations.

Not everybody, however, feels comfortable in dealing with the research requirements. A "research phobia" can be detected among college students and even some faculty members, as well as practitioners who label themselves as clinicians. If they are forced to do research and the research experience turns out to be not so positive as expected, then their nervousness about research is likely to persist. And that may seriously hurt their career opportunities. An ill-prepared researcher, in turn, can only produce poor research designs and results, which will sooner or later hurt the research undertakings.

Research, indeed, can be very challenging even to experienced researchers and professors. Yet this fact should not be interpreted to mean it would take years of classroom instruction before a student can be assigned a research task. The reality is that many students come to pursue an advanced degree, where an independent research project is a normal requirement, without sufficient research skills. But a good number of them have survived the challenges and some succeeded with their achievements in relatively short periods of time.

The success, of course, has not always been without struggles and difficulties. It is not uncommon to see students owning a number of research books without knowing how to proceed with their own projects. It is also not unusual for the students, having taken statistics courses, not to know what it really does. Good textbooks and professors are often readily available, but they do not automatically improve the students' skills. As a matter of fact, the way the students acquire research skills and the way the texts deal with the subject could be very different. Student researchers must clarify their needs and combine what is said in the texts with what is encountered in practice. A typical problem, however, is that the multihundred-page textbooks usually contain too much material that does

replacement of part or all of the old cases with the new ones as long as the selection criteria apply. Unlike the other two designs, this type of study may avoid the aging effect by always selecting samples of the same age.

The selection of a longitudinal design depends on your specific research questions, or what you need to compare along the time dimension. If you just want to compare two populations of the same type at different times, yours can be a simple trend study. If you need to compare two samples drawn in different periods from the same population, you may use a cohort design. If you have to compare a sample with itself as it changes over time, then you must have a panel design.

Experimentation is a special kind of panel design, which has a structure that is extremely important to the advancement of behavioral and social science knowledge. The terms "causation" and "explanation" are most frequently associated with the use of experimental designs. There is a feature that distinguishes an experiment from a simple panel design. In order to explain one or a few variables of interest (dependent variables), an independent variable should be manipulable and is often called a stimulus or an experimental variable. In practice, this involves action, or is regarded as an intervention, which serves as a base for it to be potentially an intensive action or intervention research. An ordinary panel study, in contrast, may just follow a natural course of change over time.

Both an ordinary panel study and an experimental design tend to involve a number of variables in the research process. The experimenter, however, must not confuse the experimental variable with all other variables that may also be called "independent variables," or more accurately "intervening variables." In practice, it is not unusual that a researcher has devised an experiment without clearly designating the stimulus or intervention. And the researcher is likely to get overwhelmed and confused by all kinds of variables she has to deal with later in implementing the design.

The basic logic of experimentation is to measure the dependent variable(s) first (called pretesting, with the result denoted by E_1), then to expose the subjects to a stimulus, or the influence of an independent variable. Then the dependent variables are re-measured (called posttesting, with the result denoted by E_2). Differences noted between the pretest and the posttest ($E_2 - E_1$) on the dependent variable now can be attributed to the influence of the independent variable.

The validity of this single group design is questionable, however. There could be many other factors that are also at work to cause change in the subjects over

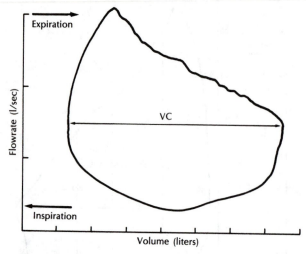

FIG 1–40.
Flow-volume loop, obstructive pattern. *VC* = vital capacity.

- Calcification (e.g., tuberculosis)
- Fibrosis (e.g., pneumoconiosis)
- Bronchogenic tumor (e.g., squamous cell carcinoma)
- Caseating tubercles (e.g., tuberculosis)
- Cavitations (e.g., tuberculosis)

The above pathologic conditions cause lung rigidity to increase. When lung rigidity increases, lung compliance decreases. Decreased lung compliance causes a reduction in the patient's VC, RV, FRC, and TLC (Fig 1–42). In addition, when lung compliance decreases, the patient's ventilatory rate commonly increases while, at the same time, the VT decreases (see Fig 1–26).

Pulmonary Function Studies: Expiratory Maneuver Findings Characteristic of Obstructive Lung Diseases

- Decreased forced vital capacity (FVC)
- Decreased forced expiratory flow 200–1,200 ($FEF_{200-1,200}$)
- Decreased forced expiratory flow 25%–75% ($FEF_{25\%-75\%}$)
- Decreased forced expiratory volume, timed (FEV_T)
- Decreased forced expiratory volume in 1 second/forced vital capacity ratio (FEV_1/FVC ratio)
- Decreased maximum voluntary ventilation (MVV)
- Decreased peak expiratory flow rate (PEFR)
- Decreased flow at 50% vital capacity ($\dot{V}_{max50}$)

The above expiratory maneuver findings develop in response to pathologic conditions that alter the anatomic structures of the tracheobronchial tree. Such pathologic conditions include the following:

- Chronic inflammation and swelling of the peripheral airways
- Excessive mucus production and accumulation

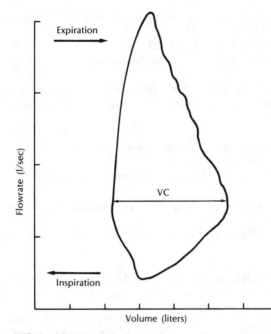

FIG 1–41.
Flow-volume loop, restrictive pattern. *VC* = vital capacity.

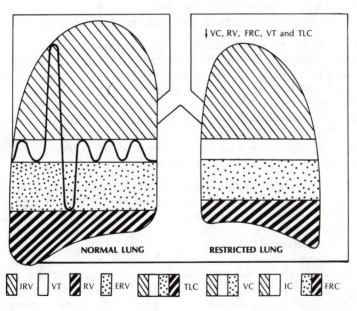

FIG 1–42.
How restrictive lung disorders alter lung volumes and capacities. *IRV* = inspiratory reserve volume; *V$_T$* = tidal volume; *RV* = residual volume; *ERV* = expiratory reserve volume; *TLC* = total lung capacity; *VC* = vital capacity; *IC* = inspiratory capacity; *FRC* = functional residual capacity.

- Bronchial airway obstruction (e.g., from mucus or from a tumor projecting into a bronchus)
- Destruction and weakening of the distal airways
- Smooth muscle constriction of the bronchial airways

To fully appreciate how the above pathologic conditions cause the expiratory maneuver findings seen in obstructive pulmonary disorders, an understanding of the following is essential:

- How activation of the dynamic compression mechanism affects respiratory function in obstructive pulmonary diseases
- Bernoulli's principle and the dynamic compression mechanism in obstructive pulmonary diseases
- How Poiseuille's law relates to respiratory function in obstructive pulmonary diseases
- How the airway resistance equation relates to respiratory function in obstructive pulmonary diseases

How Activation of the Dynamic Compression Mechanism Affects Respiratory Function in Obstructive Pulmonary Diseases.—

The effort-dependent portion of a forced expiratory maneuver.—Normally, during approximately the first 30% of a forced vital capacity maneuver, the maximum peak flow rate is dependent on the amount of muscular effort exerted by the individual. Therefore, the first 30% of a forced expiratory maneuver is referred to as effort dependent. In other words, the initial flow rate during forced expiration depends on the muscular effort produced by the individual.

The effort-independent portion of a forced expiratory maneuver.—The flow rate during approximately the last 70% of a forced vital capacity maneuver is effort independent, that is, once a maximum flow rate has been attained, the flow rate cannot be increased by further muscular effort.

The lung volume at which the patient initiates a forced expiratory maneuver also influences the maximum flow rate. As lung volumes decline, flow also declines. The reduced flow, however, is the maximum flow for that particular volume.

Figure 1–43 illustrates where the effort-dependent and effort-independent portions of a forced expiratory maneuver appear on a flow-volume loop.

Dynamic compression of the bronchial airways.—The limitation of the flow rate that occurs during approximately the last 70% of a forced vital capacity maneuver is due to the *dynamic compression* of the walls of the airways. As gas flows through the airways to the atmosphere during passive expiration, the pressure within the airways diminishes to zero (Fig 1–44,A).

During a forced expiratory maneuver, however, as the airway pressure decreases from the alveolus to the atmosphere, there comes a point at which the pressure within the lumen of the airways equals the pleural pressure surrounding the airways. The transpulmonary pressure at this point is zero. This is called the *equal-pressure point.*

Downstream (i.e., toward the mouth) from the equal-pressure point, the lateral pressure within the airway becomes less than the surrounding pleural pressure. Consequently, the airways are compressed. As muscular effort and pleural pressure increase during a forced expiratory maneuver, the equal-pressure point moves upstream (i.e., toward the alveolus). Ultimately, the equal-pressure point becomes fixed where the individual's flow rate has achieved a maximum (see Fig

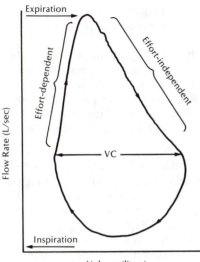
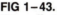

FIG 1–43.
The effort-dependent and effort-independent portions of a forced expiratory maneuver in a flow-volume loop measurement. *VC* = vital capacity.

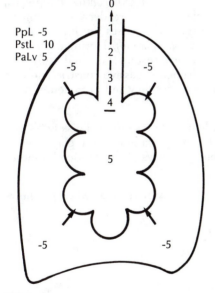
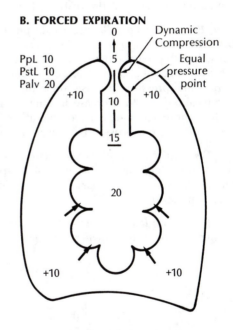

FIG 1–44.
The dynamic compression mechanism. **A,** during passive expiration, static elastic recoil pressure *(PstL)* is 10, pleural pressure *(PpL)* at the beginning of expiration is −5, and alveolar pressure *(Palv)* is +5. In order for gas to move from the alveolus to the atmosphere during expiration, the pressure must decrease progressively in the airways from +5 to 0. As **A** shows, PpL is always less than the airway pressure. **B,** during forced expiration, PpL becomes positive (+10 in this illustration). When this PpL is added to a PstL of +10, Palv becomes +20. As the pressure progressively decreases during forced expiration, there must be a point at which the pressures inside and outside the airway wall are equal. This point is the equal pressure point. Airway compression occurs downstream (toward the mouth) from this point because the lateral pressure in the lumen is less than the surrounding wall pressure.

1–44,B). In essence, once dynamic compression occurs during a forced expiratory maneuver, increased muscular effort merely augments airway compression, which in turn increases airway resistance.

As the structural changes associated with obstructive pulmonary diseases intensify, the patient commonly responds by increasing intrapleural pressure during expiration to overcome the increased airway resistance produced by the disease. By increasing intrapleural pressure during expiration, however, the patient activates the dynamic compression mechanism, which in turn further reduces the diameter of the bronchial airways. This results in an even greater increase in airway resistance.

Bernoulli's Principle and the Dynamic Compression Mechanism in Obstructive Pulmonary Diseases.—Bernoulli's principle states that when a gas flowing through a tube encounters a narrowing or restriction, the velocity of the gas molecules increases. As a result, the gas molecules collide less frequently with the sides of the tube, and this causes the lateral pressure to drop (Fig 1–45).

This mechanism may play an insidious role in certain pulmonary disorders. In chronic obstructive pulmonary disease, for example, when the gas flow encounters bronchial narrowing during a forced expiratory maneuver, the decreased lateral pressure that results at the restricted sites enhances dynamic compression.

How Poiseuille's Law Relates to Respiratory Function in Obstructive Pulmonary Diseases.—During a normal inspiration, intrapleural pressure decreases from its normal resting level (about 2 to 3 cm H_2O pressure) and causes the bronchial airways to lengthen and to increase in diameter (passive dilation). During expiration, intrapleural pressure increases (or returns to its normal resting state) and causes the bronchial airways to decrease in length and in diameter (passive constriction) (Fig 1–46). These anatomic changes can affect bronchial gas flow and intrapleural pressure and can be expressed by Poiseuille's law.

Poiseuille's law and its significance.—Although the factors in Poiseuille's law are of little significance during normal, spontaneous breathing, they play a major role in obstructive pulmonary disorders. Poiseuille's law can be expressed for either flow or pressure.

Poiseuille's law for flow.—Poiseuille's law for flow states that when gas flows through a tube, the following applies:

$$\dot{V} = \frac{\Delta P \pi r^4}{8ln}$$

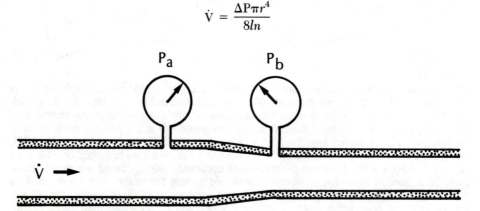

FIG 1–45.
Illustration of Bernoulli's principle.

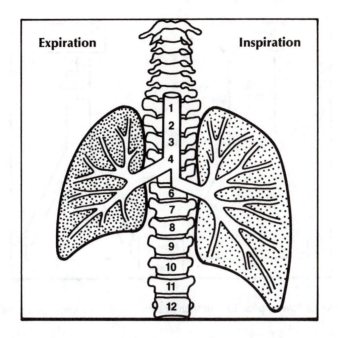

FIG 1–46.
The normal change in size of the tracheobronchial tree during inspiration and expiration.

where n is the viscosity of a gas (or fluid), ΔP is the change of pressure from one end of the tube to the other, r is the radius of the tube, l is the length of the tube, and $\dot{V}$ is the gas (or fluid) flow through the tube; π and 8 are constants that will be excluded from the present discussion.

The equation states that flow is directly related to P and r^4 and indirectly related to l and n. In other words, flow will decrease in response to a decreased P and tube radius. Flow will increase in response to a decreased tube length and viscosity. Conversely, flow will increase in response to an increased P and tube radius and decrease in response to an increased tube length and viscosity.

It should be emphasized that flow is profoundly affected by the radius of the tube. As Poiseuille's law illustrates, $\dot{V}$ is a function of the fourth power of the radius (r^4). In other words, assuming pressure (ΔP) remains constant, decreasing the radius of a tube by one half reduces the gas flow to $\frac{1}{16}$ of its original flow.

For example, if the radius of a bronchial tube through which gas flows at a rate of 16 ml/sec is reduced to one half its original size because of mucosal swelling, the flow rate through the bronchial tube would decrease to 1 mL/sec ($\frac{1}{16}$ the original flow rate) (Fig 1–47).

Similarly, decreasing a tube radius by 16% decreases gas flow to one half its original rate. For instance, if the radius of a bronchial tube through which gas flows at a rate of 16 mL/sec is decreased by 16% (because of mucosal swelling, for example), the flow rate through the bronchial tube would decrease to 8 mL/sec (one half the original flow rate) (Fig 1–48).

Poiseuille's law for pressure.—When Poiseuille's law is rearranged for pressure, it is written as follows:

$$P = \frac{\dot{V}8ln}{\pi r^4}$$

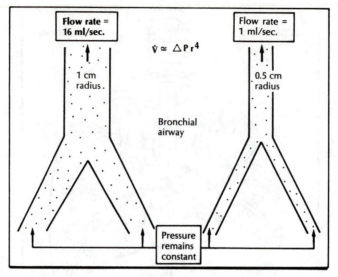

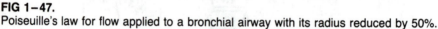

FIG 1–47.
Poiseuille's law for flow applied to a bronchial airway with its radius reduced by 50%.

The equation now states that pressure is directly related to $\dot{V}$, l, and n and indirectly related to r^4. In other words, pressure will increase in response to a decreased tube radius and decrease in response to a decreased flow rate, tube length, or viscosity. The opposite is also true: pressure will decrease in response to an increased tube radius and increase in response to an increased flow rate, tube length, or viscosity.

Pressure is a function of the radius to the fourth power and therefore is profoundly affected by the radius of a tube. In other words, if flow ($\dot{V}$) remains con-

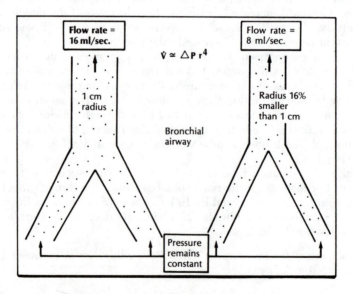

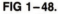

FIG 1–48.
Poiseuille's law for flow applied to a bronchial airway with its radius reduced by 16%.

stant, decreasing a tube radius to one half its previous size requires an increase in pressure to 16 times its original level.

For example, if the radius of a bronchial tube with a driving pressure of 1 cm H_2O is reduced to one half its original size because of mucosal swelling, the driving pressure through the bronchial tube would have to increase to 16 cm H_2O (16 × 1 = 16) to maintain the same flow rate (Fig 1–49).

Similarly, decreasing the tube radius by 16% increases the pressure to twice its original level. For instance, if the radius of a bronchial tube with a driving pressure of 10 cm H_2O is decreased by 16% because of mucosal swelling, the driving pressure through the bronchial tube would have to increase to 20 cm H_2O (twice its original pressure) to maintain the same flow (Fig 1–50).

Poiseuille's law rearranged to simple proportionalities.—When Poiseuille's law is applied to the tracheobronchial tree during spontaneous breathing, the two equations can be rewritten as simple proportionalities:

$$\dot{V} \simeq Pr^4 \qquad P \simeq \frac{\dot{V}}{r^4}$$

where P is the intrapleural pressure, $\dot{V}$ is gas flow through the tracheobronchial tree, and r is the radius of the bronchi.

Based upon the proportionality for flow ($\dot{V} = Pr^4$), it can be stated that since gas flow varies directly with r^4 of the bronchial airway, flow must diminish during exhalation as the radius of the bronchial airways decreases. Stated differently, assuming that the pressure remains constant as the radius (r) of the bronchial airways decreases, the gas flow ($\dot{V}$) also decreases. During normal spontaneous breathing, the gas flow reduction during exhalation is negligible.

In terms of the proportionality for pressure ($P = \dot{V}/r^4$), if the gas flow is to remain constant during exhalation, the intrapleural pressure must vary indirectly with the fourth power of the radius of the airway. In other words, as the radius of the

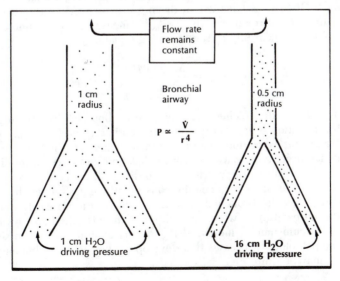

FIG 1–49.
Poiseuille's law for pressure applied to a bronchial airway with its radius reduced by 50%.

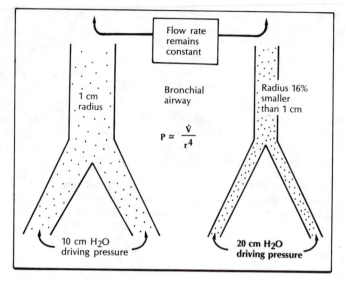

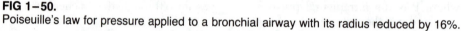

FIG 1–50.
Poiseuille's law for pressure applied to a bronchial airway with its radius reduced by 16%.

bronchial airways decreases during exhalation, the driving pressure must increase to maintain a constant gas flow. During normal spontaneous breathing, the need to increase intrapleural pressure during exhalation in order to maintain a certain gas flow is negligible.

In obstructive pulmonary diseases, however, both bronchial gas flow ($\dot{V}$) and intrapleural pressure (ΔP) may change substantially in response to the pathologic processes associated with the disorders.*

How the Airway Resistance Equation Relates to Respiratory Function in Obstructive Pulmonary Diseases.—Changes in driving pressure (ΔP) and gas flow ($\dot{V}$) are used to measure airway resistance (R_{aw}). R_{aw} is measured in centimeters of water per liter per second, according to the following equation:

$$R_{aw} = \frac{\Delta P \ (cm \ H_2O)}{\dot{V} \ (L/sec)}$$

Normally, R_{aw} in the tracheobronchial tree is about 1.0 to 2.0 cm H_2O/L/sec. When the R_{aw} equation is applied to a normal ventilatory cycle, it can be seen that R_{aw} is greater during expiration than during inspiration. This is because the radius of the bronchial airways decreases during exhalation and—as Poiseuille's law for flow demonstrates—causes the gas flow ($\dot{V}$) to diminish.

Theoretically, during normal spontaneous breathing gas enters the alveoli during inspiration (when the bronchial airways are dilated) more easily than it leaves the alveoli during expiration (when the caliber of the bronchial airways is smaller). Under normal circumstances, increased R_{aw} during expiration is of no significance. Because of the pathologic processes that develop in obstructive pulmonary diseases, however, R_{aw} may be quite high.

*See a mathematic discussion of Poiseuille's law for flow and pressure in Appendix X: Mathematics.

Pulmonary Function Studies: Lung Volume and Capacity Findings Characteristic of Obstructive Lung Diseases

- Increased tidal volume (VT)
- Increased residual volume (RV)
- Increased residual volume/total lung capacity ratio (RV/TLC)
- Increased functional residual capacity (FRC)
- Increased closing volume (CV)
- Decreased vital capacity (VC)
- Decreased inspiratory reserve volume (IRV)
- Decreased expiratory reserve volume (ERV)

The above lung volumes and capacities develop in response to pathologic conditions that alter the anatomic structures of the tracheobronchial tree:

- Chronic inflammation and swelling of the peripheral airways
- Excessive mucus production and accumulation
- Bronchial airway obstruction (e.g., from mucus or from a tumor projecting into a bronchus)
- Destruction and weakening of the distal airways
- Smooth muscle constriction of the bronchial airways

The above pathologic conditions cause increased airway resistance (R_{aw}) and bronchial closure during expiration. When R_{aw} becomes high, the patient's ventila-

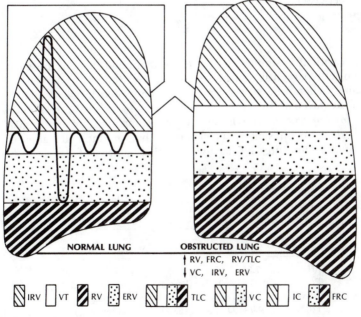

FIG 1–51.
How obstructive lung disorders alter lung volumes and capacities. *IRV* = inspiratory reserve volume; *VT* = tidal volume; *RV* = residual volume; *ERV* = expiratory reserve volume; *TLC* = total lung capacity; *VC* = vital capacity; *IC* = inspiratory capacity; *FRC* = functional residual capacity.

time. A typical problem is the effect of the experiment itself, or its "pollution" as would be termed, through the pretest-posttest process. The subjects may purposively modify or clean up their answers to the posttest based on their experience in the pretest, or simply respond to the attention they receive during the experiment. Due to such impacts, single-group study can only be considered a kind of quasi-experimental design. To rule out such influences, you need to apply some sort of control, which is the central idea in any explanatory research. An experimental design is actually used as an effective way to apply control (called experimental control, as opposed to statistical control that will be discussed later). This is done by dividing the sample into two groups, i.e., the experimental group and the control group. The two groups are supposed to be equal except that the experimental group will be exposed to the stimulus or intervention while the control group will not. This difference can be concealed, for example, by giving the control group merely a placebo (such as a sugar pill) in a new drug trial. To avoid observational bias on the part of the researcher, the observer may not be told either about which subject belongs to which group. Both groups go through the same pretest-posttest process and are subject to any change (inside or outside the experiment) over the experimental period, except that caused by the intervention. Subtracting the average effect of change in the control group ($C = C_2 - C_1$) from that in the experimental group $E = (E_2 - E_1)$, therefore, will give the net effect brought about by the stimulus or the intervention. That is, net effect $= E - C = (E_2 - E_1) - (C_2 - C_1) = (E_2 - C_2) - (E_1 - C_1)$.

Note, if the experimental group and the control group are really the same, then the pretest results will be equal for both groups (i.e., $E_1 = C_1$) and the net effect of the intervention will be simply determined by the posttest results (i.e., $E_2 - C_2$). In other words, the pretesting of both groups is not needed. This is actually a strategy we will see later to avoid some negative effect of the pretesting procedure. The problem is, even random assignment of subjects does not guarantee with a hundred percent confidence that the two groups will be exactly the same. Therefore, a posttest-only study is usually regarded as another kind of quasi-experimental design.

Like any panel design, an important issue facing experimental research is to select a representative sample and maintain its representativeness during the entire period of study. This is an issue concerning the external validity or generalizability of the experiment. Here, the problem of panel attrition takes the form of experimental mortality, referring to the dropping out of subjects before an experiment is completed. This would result in selection bias and thus distort

tory rate commonly decreases while, at the same time, the VT increases. This ventilatory pattern is thought to be adopted to reduce the work of breathing (see Fig 1–26).

When bronchial closure develops during expiration, gas that enters the alveoli during inspiration, when the bronchi are naturally wider, is prevented from leaving the alveoli during expiration. The alveoli then become overdistended with gas, a condition known as air trapping. Thus, excluding the VT, bronchial closure and air trapping are the major mechanisms responsible for the abnormal lung volume and capacity findings seen in obstructive pulmonary diseases (Fig 1–51).

Common Abnormal Arterial Blood Gas Findings in Respiratory Diseases

As the pathologic processes of a respiratory disorder intensify, the patient's arterial blood gas values are usually altered to some degree. Table 1–5 lists the normal arterial blood gas values. Common abnormal arterial blood gases associated with respiratory diseases are (1) *acute alveolar hyperventilation with hypoxemia*, (2) *acute ventilatory failure with hypoxemia*, and (3) *chronic ventilatory failure with hypoxemia*.

Acute Alveolar Hyperventilation With Hypoxemia

- Pa_{O_2}: decreased
- Pa_{CO_2}: decreased
- HCO_3^-: decreased
- pH: increased

When a patient is stimulated to breathe more and has the muscular power to do so, alveolar hyperventilation may develop, i.e., the Pa_{CO_2} decreases below the normal value. When a decreased Pa_{CO_2} is accompanied by alkalemia (a pH above normal), acute alveolar hyperventilation is said to exist. In respiratory disease, *acute alveolar hyperventilation* is commonly accompanied by hypoxemia.

The basic pathophysiologic mechanisms that produce the abnormal arterial blood gas findings in acute alveolar hyperventilation are as follows:

TABLE 1–5.
Normal Blood Gas Values

Blood Gas Value*	Arterial	Venous
pH	7.35–7.45	7.30–7.40
P_{CO_2}	35–45 mm Hg (Pa_{CO_2})	42–48 mm Hg ($P\bar{v}_{CO_2}$)
HCO_3^-	22–28 mEq/L	24–30 mEq/L
Po_2	80–100 mm Hg (Pa_{O_2})	35–45 mm Hg ($P\bar{v}_{O_2}$)

*Technically, only the oxygen (P_{O_2}) and carbon dioxide (P_{CO_2}) pressure readings are "true" blood gas values. The pH indicates the balance between the bases and acids in the blood. The bicarbonate (HCO_3^-) reading is an indirect measurement that is calculated from the pH and P_{CO_2} levels.

Decreased Pa$_{O_2}$, Decreased Pa$_{CO_2}$.—The decreased Pa$_{O_2}$ seen during acute alveolar hyperventilation most commonly develops from the decreased $\dot{V}/\dot{Q}$ ratio, capillary shunting (or a shuntlike effect), and venous admixture associated with the pulmonary disorder. The Pa$_{O_2}$ will continue to drop as the pathologic effects of the disease intensify. Eventually, the Pa$_{O_2}$ may decline to a point low enough (a Pa$_{O_2}$ of about 60 mm Hg) to stimulate the peripheral chemoreceptors, which in turn causes the ventilatory rate to increase (Fig 1–52). Once this happens, the patient's Pa$_{O_2}$ generally remains at a constant level. The increased ventilatory response, however, is often accompanied by a decline in the Pa$_{CO_2}$ (Fig 1–53).

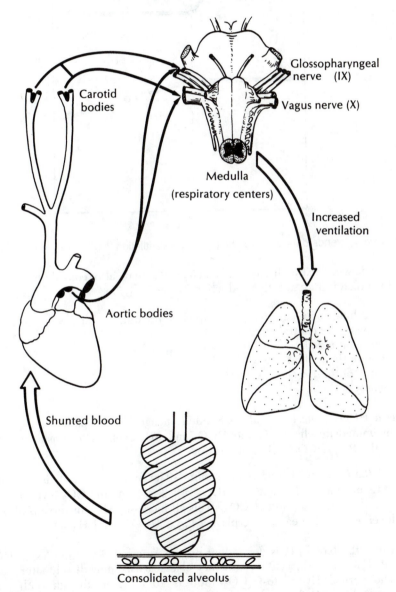

FIG 1–52.
Relationship of venous admixture to stimulation of peripheral chemoreceptors in response to alveolar consolidation.

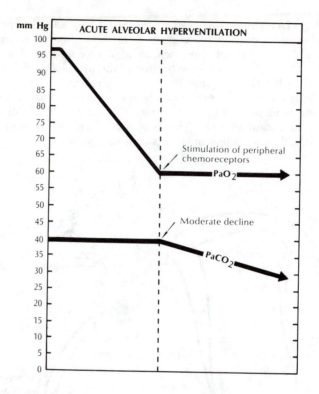

FIG 1–53.
Pa_{O_2} and Pa_{CO_2} trends during acute alveolar hyperventilation.

The following pathophysiologic mechanisms may also contribute to an increased ventilatory rate and to a reduction in the Pa_{CO_2}*:

- Decreased lung compliance/increased work of breathing relationship
- Stimulation of the central chemoreceptors
- Activation of the deflation reflex
- Activation of the irritant reflex
- Stimulation of the J receptors
- Pain/anxiety

Decreased HCO_3^-, **Increased pH.**—Sudden changes in the patient's Pa_{CO_2} level cause an immediate change in the HCO_3^- and pH levels. The reason for this is based on the $P_{CO_2}/HCO_3^-/pH$ relationship.

Review of the $P_{CO_2}/HCO_3^-/pH$ **relationship.**—The bulk of the CO_2 is transported from the tissue cells to the lungs as HCO_3^- (Fig 1–54). As the CO_2 level increases, the plasma P_{CO_2}, HCO_3^-, and H_2CO_3 levels all increase. The converse is also true: as the level of CO_2 decreases, the plasma P_{CO_2}, HCO_3^-, and H_2CO_3 levels all decrease.

Because the blood pH is dependent on the ratio between the plasma HCO_3^- (base) and H_2CO_3 (acid), acute ventilatory changes will immediately alter the pH level. The normal HCO_3^--to-H_2CO_3 ratio is 20:1. Even though both plasma HCO_3^- and plasma H_2CO_3 move in the same direction during acute ventilatory

*See the section on increased respiratory rate, page 23.

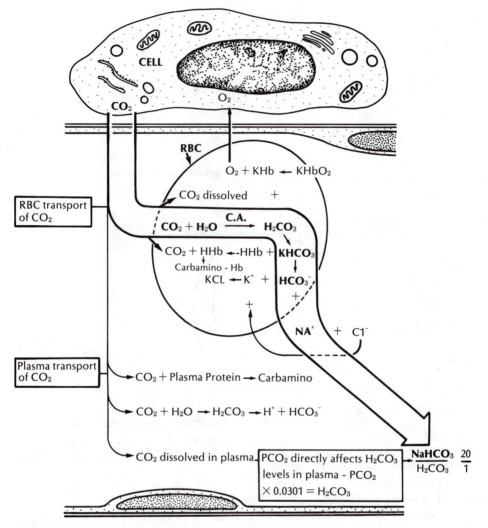

FIG 1–54.
Transportation of CO_2 in the form of HCO_3^- from the tissue cells to the lungs. *CA* = carbonic anhydrase.

changes, acute changes in the H_2CO_3 level play a much more powerful role in altering the pH status than do acute changes in the HCO_3^- level. This is due to the 20:1 ratio between HCO_3^- to H_2CO_3.

In other words, for every H_2CO_3 molecule increase or decrease, 20 HCO_3^- molecules must also increase or decrease, respectively. If this does not happen, the normal 20:1 ratio between the HCO_3^- and H_2CO_3 will change. When the HCO_3^--to-H_2CO_3 ratio is less than 20:1, an *acidic* condition exists. When the HCO_3^--to-H_2CO_3 ratio is greater than 20:1, an *alkalotic* condition exists.

In view of the above relationship, during periods of acute alveolar hyperventilation the $P_{A_{CO_2}}$ will decrease and allow more CO_2 to leave the pulmonary blood. This action necessarily decreases the blood P_{CO_2}, H_2CO_3, and HCO_3^- levels (Fig 1–55). Because acute changes in H_2CO_3 levels are more significant than are acute changes in HCO_3^- levels, an increased HCO_3^--to-H_2CO_3 ratio develops (a ratio

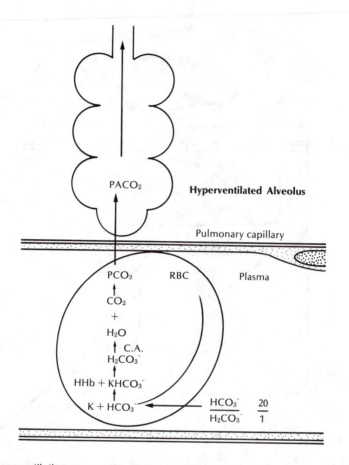

FIG 1–55.
Alveolar hyperventilation causes the $P_{A_{CO_2}}$, and the plasma P_{CO_2}, HCO_3^-, and H_2CO_3 to all decrease. *CA* = carbonic anhydrase.

greater than 20:1). This action causes the patient's blood pH to increase, or become more alkaline. The normal buffer line on the $PCO_2/HCO_3^-/pH$ nomogram in Figure 1–56 illustrates the expected HCO_3^- and pH changes that develop in response to sudden CO_2 changes only.

Acute Ventilatory Failure With Hypoxemia

- Pa_{O_2}: Decreased
- Pa_{CO_2}: Increased
- HCO_3^-: Increased
- pH: Decreased

Ventilatory failure is defined as a condition in which the lungs are unable to meet the metabolic demands of the body in terms of carbon dioxide homeostasis. In other words, the patient is unable to provide the muscular, mechanical work necessary to move gas into and out of the lungs to meet the carbon dioxide metabolic demands of the body. This condition leads to an increased $P_{A_{CO_2}}$ and, subsequently, to an increased Pa_{CO_2} level. Ventilatory failure is not associated with a

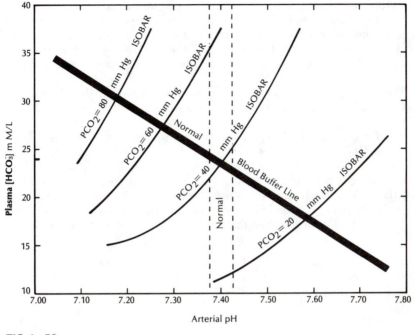

FIG 1–56.
$P_{CO_2}/HCO_3^-/pH$ relationship.

"typical ventilatory pattern." The patient may by apneic or have severe hyperpnea and tachypnea. The bottom line is that ventilatory failure will develop in response to any ventilatory pattern that is not sufficient in terms of alveolar ventilation. When an increased Pa_{CO_2} is accompanied by acidemia (decreased pH), *acute ventilatory failure* is said to exist. Clinically, this is a medical emergency, and mechanical ventilation is indicated.

The basic pathophysiologic mechanisms that produce the abnormal arterial blood gas findings in acute ventilatory failure are as follows.

Decreased Pa_{O_2}, Increased Pa_{CO_2}.—Whenever a respiratory disorder becomes critical over a relatively short period of time, acute ventilatory failure may develop. When this happens, the patient's overall $\dot{V}/\dot{Q}$ ratio decreases. This condition causes the PA_{O_2} to decrease and the PA_{CO_2} to increase. This action in turn causes the Pa_{O_2} to decrease and the Pa_{CO_2} to increase.

Increased HCO_3^-, Decreased pH.—The sudden rise in the Pa_{CO_2} level causes the H_2CO_3 and HCO_3^- levels to increase (Fig 1–57). Because acute changes in H_2CO_3 are more significant than acute changes in HCO_3^- are, a decreased HCO_3^--to-H_2CO_3 ratio develops (a ratio less than 20:1). This action causes the patient's blood pH to decrease, or become less alkaline.

Chronic Ventilatory Failure With Hypoxemia

- Pa_{O_2}: decreased
- Pa_{CO_2}: increased
- HCO_3^-: increased
- pH: normal

   Chronic ventilatory failure is defined as a greater-than-normal Pa_{CO_2} level with a normal pH status. Clinically, the chronic hypercarbia is most commonly seen in severe chronic obstructive pulmonary disease. Chronic ventilatory failure, however, is seen in other respiratory diseases. Table 1–6 lists some respiratory diseases associated with chronic ventilatory failure during the advanced stages of the disorder.
   The basic pathophysiologic mechanisms that produce the abnormal arterial blood gas findings in chronic ventilatory failure are as follows.

Decreased Pa_{O_2}, Increased Pa_{CO_2}.—When a respiratory disorder becomes critical over a relatively long period of time (e.g., chronic bronchitis or emphysema), the work of breathing may become so great and the pulmonary shunting so significant that more oxygen is consumed than is gained. Although the exact mechanism is unclear, the patient slowly develops a breathing pattern that uses the least amount of oxygen for the energy expended. In essence, the patient selects a breathing pattern based on work efficiency rather than ventilatory efficiency.* As a result, the pa-

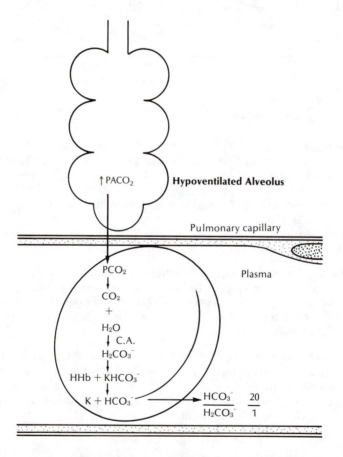

FIG 1–57.
Alveolar hypoventilation causes the $P_{A_{CO_2}}$, and the plasma P_{CO_2}, HCO_3^-, and H_2CO_3 to all increase. CA = carbonic anhydrase.

---

*See the discussion on how lung compliance and airway resistance affect ventilatory patterns, page 24.

TABLE 1–6.
Respiratory Diseases Associated With Chronic
Ventilatory Failure During the Advanced Stages

Chronic Obstructive Pulmonary Diseases (Most Common)	Other Respiratory Diseases
Chronic bronchitis	Pneumoconiosis
Emphysema	Tuberculosis
Bronchiectasis	Fungal diseases
Cystic fibrosis	Kyphoscoliosis

tient's alveolar ventilation slowly decreases, which in turn causes the Pa_{O_2} to decrease and the Pa_{CO_2} to increase (Fig 1–58).

Increased HCO_3^-, *Normal pH*.—When an individual hypoventilates for a long period of time, the kidneys will try to correct the decreased pH by retaining HCO_3^- in the blood. Renal compensation in the presence of chronic hypoventilation can be shown when the calculated HCO_3^- and pH readings are higher than expected for a particular P_{CO_2} level. For example, in terms of the absolute $P_{CO_2}/HCO_3^-/pH$ relationship, when the P_{CO_2} level is about 80 mm Hg, the HCO_3^- level should be about 30 mM/L, and the pH should be about 7.19, according to the normal blood buffer line (Fig 1–59). If the HCO_3^- and pH levels are greater than these values (i.e., the pH and HCO_3^- readings cross a P_{CO_2} isobar* above the normal blood buffer line in the upper left-hand corner of the nomogram), renal retention of HCO_3^- (partial renal compensation) has likely occurred. When the HCO_3^- level increases enough to return the acidic pH to normal, complete renal compensation is said to have occurred (chronic ventilatory failure).

As a general rule, the kidneys do not overcompensate for an abnormal pH level, that is, should the patient's blood pH level become acidic for a long period of time due to hypoventilation, the kidneys will not retain enough HCO_3^- for the pH value to climb higher than 7.4. The opposite is also true: should the patient's blood pH become alkalotic for a long period of time due to hyperventilation, the kidneys will not excrete enough HCO_3^- to cause the pH level to fall below 7.4.

In persons who have been hypoventilating over a long period of time, however, it is not uncommon to find a pH level greater than 7.4. This is believed to be due to the water and chloride ion shifts between the intracellular and extracellular spaces that occur while the kidneys are compensating for a decreased blood pH.

To summarize, the lungs play an important role in maintaining the P_{CO_2}, HCO_3^-, and pH levels on a moment-to-moment basis. The kidneys, on the other hand, play an important role in maintaining the HCO_3^- and pH levels during long periods of hyperventilation or hypoventilation. It is a common error to assume that the maintenance of HCO_3^- levels in the body is solely under the influence of the kidneys.

Finally, it should be noted that modern blood gas analyzers do not provide the expected HCO_3^- and pH levels for a particular Pa_{CO_2} level. Because of this, a nomogram such as the one shown in Figure 1–56 must be used to clinically determine the expected HCO_3^- and pH values for a particular Pa_{CO_2} level.

*The isobars on the $PCO_2/HCO_3^-/pH$ nomogram illustrate the pH changes that develop in the blood as a result of (1) metabolic changes (i.e., HCO_3^- changes), or (2) a combination of metabolic and respiratory (CO_2) changes.

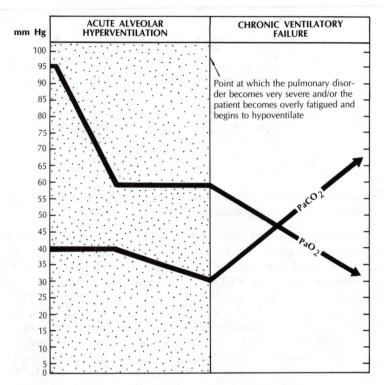

FIG 1–58.
Pa_{O_2} and Pa_{CO_2} trends during chronic ventilatory failure.

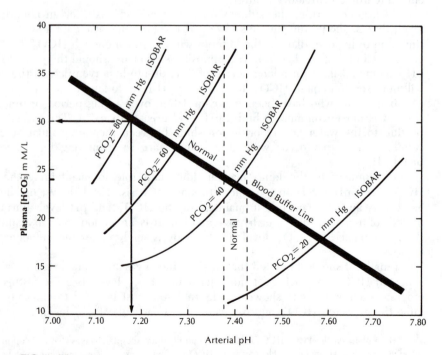

FIG 1–59.
Expected pH and HCO_3^- levels when the Pa_{CO_2} is about 80 mm Hg.

Lactic Acidosis

The nomogram shown in Figure 1–56 can also be used to indentify the possible presence of other acids or bases in the blood that are not related to either the Pa_{CO_2} level or kidney compensation. For example, when the oxygen level is inadequate to meet tissue needs (e.g., during acute or chronic ventilatory failure), alternate biochemical reactions are used that do not utilize oxygen. This is known as the anaerobic (non–oxygen-utilizing) metabolism. Lactic acid is the end product of this process. Thus, when a patient demonstrates both a reduced Pa_{O_2} level and a decreased pH value, lactic acidosis may be present. The presence of lactic acidosis is verified when the calculated HCO_3^- reading and pH level are both lower than expected for a particular Pa_{CO_2} level in terms of the absolute $P_{CO_2}/HCO_3^-/pH$ relationship.

Increased Heart Rate, Cardiac Output, and Blood Pressure

An increased heart rate, increased cardiac output, and elevated blood pressure develop frequently in pulmonary disease. This can be due to the indirect response of the heart to the hypoxic stimulation of the peripheral chemoreceptors, primarily the carotid bodies. When the carotid bodies are stimulated, reflex signals are sent to the respiratory muscles, which results in an increased rate of breathing. The increased rate of lung inflation in turn activates the so-called *pulmonary reflex*, which triggers tachycardia and an increased cardiac output and blood pressure. The increased cardiac output is a compensatory mechanism that effectively counteracts the hypoxemia produced by the shunting effects of pulmonary disorders.

This process is perhaps best understood by assuming that the body's oxygen utilization remains relatively constant over a period of time. When the cardiac output increases during a period of steady metabolic requirements, the amount of oxygen extracted from each 100 mL of blood decreases. This results in an increase in the oxygen tension of the returning venous blood, which in turn reduces the hypoxemia produced by the shunted blood. In other words, venous blood that perfuses underventilated alveoli will have less of a shunt effect if the oxygen content of the venous blood is 13 vol% as compared with, say, 10 vol%. Finally, it should be noted that when the heart rate increases beyond 150 to 175 beats per minute, cardiac output and blood pressure begin to decline.

Increased Central Venous Pressure/Decreased Systemic Blood Pressure

In patients with a severe flail chest, pneumothorax, or pleural effusion, the major veins of the chest that return blood to the right heart may be compressed. When this happens, venous return decreases, and the central venous pressure (CVP) increases. This condition is manifested by distended neck veins. The reduced venous return may also cause the patient's cardiac output and systemic pressure to decrease.

the research results. Usually the longer the experimental period, the more severe the mortality problem, which may even invalidate the entire experimental design. And the usual remedy of additional sampling may not help to save the design since the replacement cases would bring in too many variables that are out of control. A possible solution to this problem is to first include all such backup cases in a larger random sample. Then the initial study sample of the designed size as well as the replacement cases needed later can all be randomly drawn from this larger and original random sample. By including the potential replacement cases in the original, larger random sample, all their variables are put under control, although the multistage sampling technique might increase the sampling error to certain degree.

Some authors do not consider probability sampling as necessary for an experimental design, especially when it is used for the purpose of theoretical exploration. A major reason is that a social experiment seldom involves a large number of subjects in either the experimental or the control group. Probably, these authors are talking about some psychological or biological experiments. Here usually a small number of subjects are recruited from a large population that cannot be considered very heterogeneous in the aspects to be tested. This is not the case for some large-scale social experiments, however. In one of the welfare reform research projects sponsored by the State of California called the Work Pays Demonstration Project (WPDP), for example, the experimental group included 10,000 cases and the control group 5,000 cases. And the research targets, i.e., the welfare recipients, by no means could be considered a homogeneous population in terms of their social situations and economic behaviors.

Generally speaking, random sampling is still a major means to achieve the external validity of an experimental design, though the research treatment itself may be another source of problems. Campbell and Stanley (1963) identified four kinds of issues associated with the special treatment of experimentation, that is, interaction of selection bias and experimental variable, reactive effect of arrangements, reactive effect of testing, and multiple-treatment interference. There are some experimental designs that are able to address some of the problems, such as the posttest-only design mentioned above as well as more complicated Solomon four-group design in avoiding or detecting the reactive effect of pretesting.

A special issue associated with experimentation is how to divide the subjects into two different groups. This has a heavy bearing on the internal validity of the

Cough, Sputum Production, and Hemoptysis

Cough

A cough is the sudden, audible expulsion of air from the lungs and is very common in respiratory diseases, especially in disorders that cause inflammation of the tracheobronchial tree. In general, a cough is preceded by (1) a deep inspiration, (2) partial closure of the glottis, and (3) forceful contraction of the accessory muscles of expiration to expel air from the lungs. In essence, a cough is a protective mechanism that serves to clear the lungs, bronchi, or trachea of irritants and secretion. A cough also serves to prevent the aspiration of foreign materials into the lung. The effectiveness of a cough depends largely on (1) the depth of the preceding inspiration and (2) the extent of dynamic compression on the airways (see Fig 1–44,B).

A cough may be initiated voluntarily or, to some extent, suppressed voluntarily. Under most circumstances, however, a cough is a reflex that arises from stimulation of the cough or irritant receptors (also called subepithelial mechanoreceptors), which are located in the pharynx, larynx, trachea, and large bronchi. When stimulated, the irritant receptors send a signal by way of the glossopharyngeal (cranial nerve IX) and vagus (cranial nerve X) nerves to the cough reflex center located in the medulla. The medulla in turn causes the glottis to close and the accessory muscles of expiration to contract.

Some factors that stimulate the irritant receptors are as follows:

- Inflammation
- Mucus accumulation
- Noxious gases (e.g., cigarette smoke)
- Chemical inhalation
- Very hot or very cold air
- Mechanical stimulation (e.g., endotracheal suctioning, or compression of the airways).

Sputum Production

Excessive sputum production is commonly seen in respiratory diseases that cause an acute or chronic inflammation of the tracheobronchial tree (Fig 1–60).

Histology of the Tracheobronchial Tree.—The wall of the tracheobronchial tree is composed of three major layers: an epithelial lining, the lamina propria, and a cartilaginous layer (Fig 1–61).

The *epithelial lining*, which is separated from the lamina propria by a basement membrane, is predominantly composed of pseudostratified, ciliated, columnar epithelium interspersed with numerous mucus- and serum-secreting glands. The ciliated cells extend from the beginning of the trachea to—and sometimes including—the respiratory bronchioles. As the tracheobronchial tree becomes progressively smaller, the columnar structure of the ciliated cells gradually decreases in height. In the terminal bronchioles the epithelium appears more cuboidal than columnar. These cells flatten even more in the respiratory bronchioles (see Fig 1–61).

A mucous layer, commonly referred to as the mucous blanket, covers the epithelial lining of the tracheobronchial tree (Fig 1–62). The viscosity of the mucous layer progressively increases from the epithelial lining to the inner luminal surface, and there are two distinct layers: (1) the sol layer, which is adjacent to the epithelial lining, and (2) the gel layer, which is the more viscous layer adjacent to the inner luminal surface. The mucous blanket is 95% water. The remaining 5% consists of

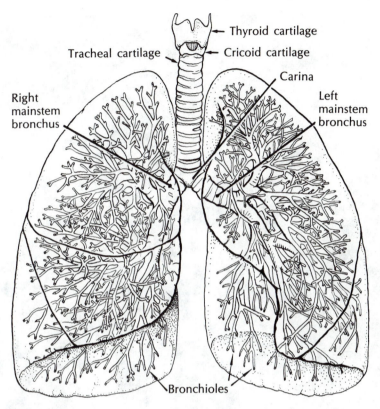

FIG 1–60.
The tracheobronchial tree.

glycoproteins, carbohydrates, lipids, DNA, some cellular debris, and foreign particles.

The mucous blanket is produced by (1) the goblet cells and (2) the submucosal, or bronchial, glands. The goblet cells are located intermittently between the pseudostratified, ciliated, columnar cells and have been identified as low as the terminal bronchioles.

Most of the mucous blanket is produced by the submucosal glands, which extend deeply into the lamina propria and are composed of several different cell types: serous cells, mucous cells, collecting duct cells, mast cells, myoepithelial cells, and clear cells, which are probably lymphocytes. The submucosal glands are particularly numerous in the medium-sized bronchi and disappear in the bronchioles. These glands are innervated by parasympathetic (cholinergic) nerve fibers and produce about 100 mL of bronchial secretions per day.

The mucous blanket is an important cleansing mechanism of the tracheobronchial tree. Inhaled particles impact and stick to the mucus. The distal ends of the cilia continually strike the innermost portion of the gel layer and propel the mucous layer, along with any foreign particles, toward the larynx. At this point, the cough mechanism moves secretions beyond the larynx and into the oropharynx. This mucociliary mechanism is commonly referred to as the mucociliary transport or the mucociliary escalator. It is estimated that the cilia move the mucous blanket at an average rate of 2 cm/min.

The submucosal layer of the tracheobronchial tree is the *lamina propria*. Within the lamina propria is a loose, fibrous tissue that contains tiny blood vessels,

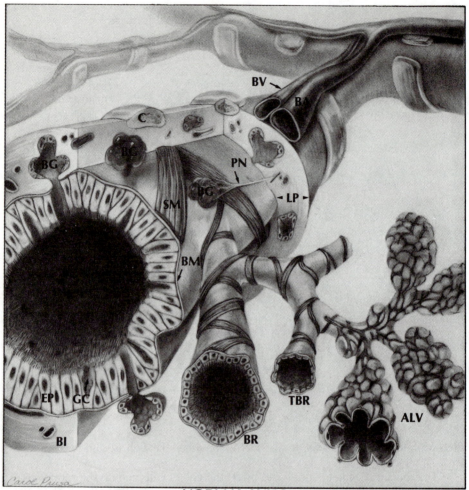

NORMAL LUNG

FIG 1–61.
The normal lung. *BG* = bronchial glands; *C* = cartilage; *BV* = bronchial vein; *BA* = bronchial artery; *SM* = smooth muscle; *PN* = parasympathetic nerve; *LP* = lamina propria; *BM* = basement membrane; *EP* = epithelium; *GC* = goblet cell; *BI* = bronchi; *BR* = bronchioles; *TBR* = terminal bronchioles; *ALV* = alveoli.

lymphatic vessels, and branches of the vagus nerve. A circular layer of smooth muscle is also found within the lamina propria. It extends from the trachea down to and including the terminal bronchioles (see Fig 1–1).

The *cartilaginous* structures that surround the tracheobronchial tree progressively diminish in size as the airways extend into the lungs. The cartilaginous layer is completely absent in bronchioles less than 1 mm in diameter (see Fig 1–61).

Types of Sputum Production.—Depending on the severity of the respiratory disease, sputum production may take several forms. For example, during the early stages of tracheobronchial tree inflammation, the sputum is usually clear, thin, and odorless. As the disease intensifies, the sputum becomes yellow-green and opaque. The yellow-green appearance results from an enzyme (myeloperoxidase) that is re-

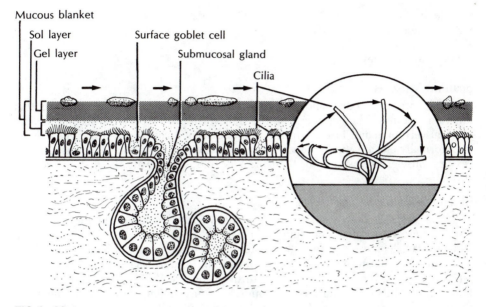

Mucous blanket
Sol layer
Gel layer
Surface goblet cell
Submucosal gland
Cilia

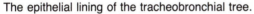

FIG 1–62.
The epithelial lining of the tracheobronchial tree.

leased during the cellular breakdown of leukocytes. It should be noted that it is possible that the yellow-green color may be caused by the expectoration of (1) retained or stagnant secretions or (2) secretions caused by an acute infection.

Thick and tenacious sputum is commonly seen in patients suffering from chronic bronchitis, bronchiectasis, cystic fibrosis, and asthma. Patients with pulmonary edema commonly expectorate a thin, frothy, pinkish sputum. Technically, this fluid is not true sputum. It results from the movement of plasma and red blood cells across the alveolar-capillary membrane into the alveoli.

Hemoptysis

Hemoptysis is the coughing up of blood or blood-tinged sputum from the tracheobronchial tree. In true hemoptysis, the sputum is usually bright red and frothy with air bubbles. Clinically, hemoptysis may be confused with hematemesis, which is blood that originates from the gastrointestinal tract and usually has a dark, coffee-ground appearance.

The repeated expectoration of blood-streaked sputum is associated with chronic bronchitis, bronchiectasis, cystic fibrosis, pulmonary embolism, lung cancer, necrotizing infections, tuberculosis, and fungal diseases.

Massive hemoptysis is defined as coughing up 400 to 600 mL of blood within a 24-hour period.

Use of the Accessory Muscles During Inspiration

During the advanced stages of chronic obstructive pulmonary disease, the accessory muscles of inspiration are activated when the diaphragm becomes significantly depressed by the increased residual volume and functional residual capacity associated with the disease. The accessory muscles assist or largely replace the diaphragm in creating a subatmospheric pressure in the lungs during inspiration. The major accessory muscles of inspiration are the following:

- Scalene muscles
- Sternocleidomastoid muscles
- Pectoralis major muscles
- Trapezius muscles

Scalene Muscles

The anterior, medial, and posterior scalene muscles are separate muscles that function as a unit. They originate on the transverse processes of the second to sixth cervical vertebrae and insert into the first and second ribs (Fig 1–63). These muscles normally elevate the first and second ribs and flex the neck. When used as accessory muscles for inspiration, their primary role is to elevate the first and second ribs.

Sternocleidomastoid Muscles

The sternocleidomastoid muscles are located on each side of the neck (Fig 1–64) where they rotate and support the head. They originate from the sternum and the clavicle and insert into the mastoid process and occipital bone of the skull.

Normally the sternocleidomastoid pulls from its sternoclavicular origin and rotates the head to the opposite side and turns it upward. When the sternocleidomastoid muscle functions as an accessory muscle of inspiration, the head and neck are fixed by other muscles, and the sternocleidomastoid pulls from its insertion on the skull and elevates the sternum. This action increases the anteroposterior diameter of the chest.

Pectoralis Major Muscles

The pectoralis majors are powerful, fan-shaped muscles that originate from the clavicle and the sternum and insert into the upper part of the humerus. The primary function of the pectoralis muscles is to pull the upper part of the arm to the body in a hugging motion (Fig 1–65).

When operating as an accessory muscle of inspiration, the pectoralis pulls from

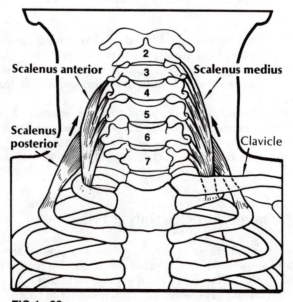

FIG 1–63.
The scalene muscle.

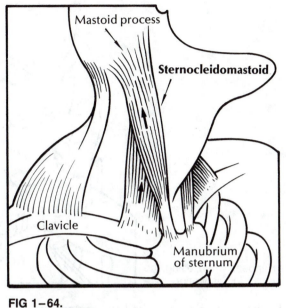

FIG 1–64.
The sternocleidomastoid muscle.

the humeral insertion and elevates the chest, thereby resulting in an increased anteroposterior diameter. It is common to observe chronic obstructive pulmonary disease patients securing their arms to something stationary and using the pectoralis major to increase the anteroposterior diameter of the chest (Fig 1–66).

Trapezius Muscles

The trapezius is a large, flat, triangular muscle that is situated superficially in the upper part of the back and the back of the neck. The muscle originates from the

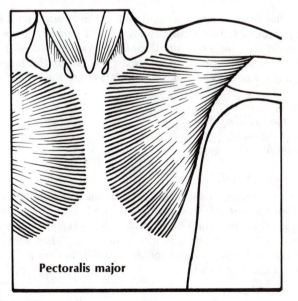

FIG 1–65.
The pectoralis major muscles.

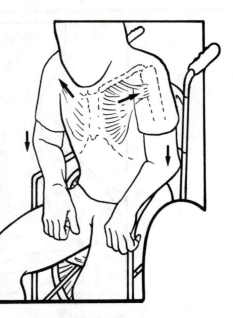

FIG 1–66.
How a patient may appear when using the
pectoralis major muscles for inspiration.

occipital bone, the ligamentum nuchae, and the spinous processes of the seventh
cervical vertebra and all the thoracic vertebrae. The muscle inserts into the spine of
the scapula, the acromion process, and the lateral third of the clavicle (Fig 1–67).
The trapezius muscle acts to rotate the scapula, raise the shoulders, and abduct and
flex the arm. Its action is typified in shrugging the shoulders (Fig 1–68).

When used as an accessory muscle of inspiration, the trapezius helps to elevate
the thoracic cage.

Use of Accessory Muscles During Expiration

Because of the airway narrowing and collapse associated with chronic obstructive pulmonary disorders, the accessory muscles of exhalation are often recruited
when airway resistance becomes significantly elevated. When these muscles ac-
tively contract, intrapleural pressure increases and offsets the increased airway resistance. The major accessory muscles of exhalation are the following:

• Rectus abdominis muscle
• External oblique muscle
• Internal oblique muscle
• Transversus abdominis muscle

Rectus Abdominis Muscle

A pair of rectus abdominis muscles extends the entire length of the abdomen.
Each muscle forms a vertical mass about 4 in. wide and is separated by the linea
alba. The muscle arises from the iliac crest and pubic symphysis and inserts into the
xyphoid process and the fifth, sixth, and seventh ribs. When activated, the muscle
assists in compressing the abdominal contents, which in turn pushes the diaphragm
into the thoracic cage (Fig 1–69).

External Oblique Muscle

The broad, thin, external oblique muscle is positioned on the anterolateral side
of the abdomen. The muscle is the longest and most superficial of all the anterolat-

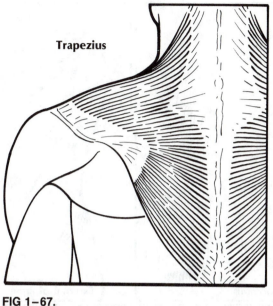

FIG 1–67.
The trapezius muscles.

eral muscles of the abdomen. It arises by eight digitations from the lower eight ribs and the abdominal aponeurosis. It inserts in the iliac crest and into the linea alba. The muscle assists in compressing the contents of the abdomen. This action also pushes the diaphragm into the thoracic cage (see Fig 1–69).

Internal Oblique Muscle

The internal oblique muscle is located in the lateral and ventral part of the abdominal wall directly under the external oblique muscle. It is smaller and thinner

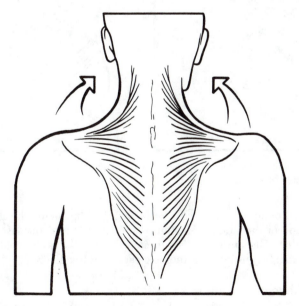

FIG 1–68.
The action of the trapezius muscle is typified in shrugging the shoulders.

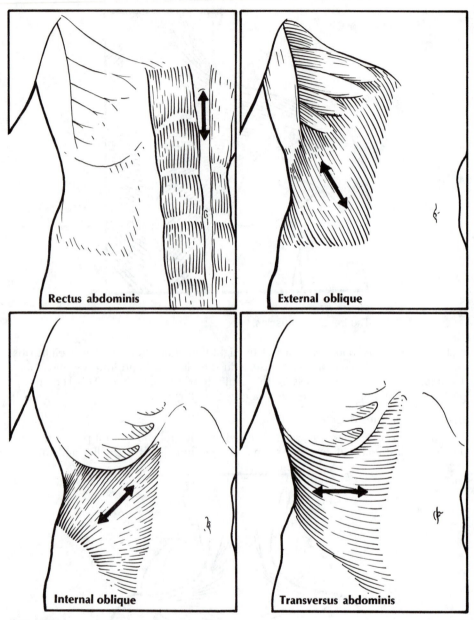

FIG 1–69.
Accessory muscles of expiration.

than the external oblique. It arises from the inguinal ligament, the iliac crest, and the lower portion of the lumbar aponeurosis. It inserts into the last four ribs and into the linea alba. The muscle assists in compressing the abdominal contents and in pushing the diaphragm into the thoracic cage (see Fig 1–69).

Transversus Abdominis Muscle

The transversus abdominis muscle is found immediately under each internal oblique muscle. The muscle arises from the inguinal ligament, the iliac crest, the thoracolumbar fascia, and the lower six ribs. It inserts into the linea alba. When activated, it also serves to constrict the abdominal contents (see Fig 1–69).

When all four pairs of accessory muscles of exhalation contract, the abdominal pressure increases and drives the diaphragm into the thoracic cage. As the diaphragm moves into the thoracic cage during exhalation, the intrapleural pressure increases and enhances the amount of gas flow (Fig 1–70).

Increased Anteroposterior Chest Diameter (Barrel Chest)

Because of the air trapping and lung hyperinflation associated with obstructive pulmonary diseases, the natural tendency of the lungs to recoil is decreased, and the normal tendency of the chest to move outward prevails. This condition results in an increased anteroposterior chest diameter and is referred to as "barrel chest." Normally, the anteroposterior chest diameter is about half the lateral diameter, or a 1:2 ratio. When the patient has a barrel chest, the ratio may be 1:1. It should be noted that the anteroposterior diameter commonly increases with aging. Thus, older individuals may have a barrel chest in the absence of any pulmonary disease. Normal newborn infants also usually have a 1:1 ratio (Fig 1–71).

Pursed-Lip Breathing

Pursed-lip breathing is commonly seen in patients during the advanced stages of obstructive pulmonary disease. It is a relatively simple technique that many patients learn without formal instruction. While pursed-lip breathing, the patient exhales through lips that are in a position similar to that of whistling, kissing, or blowing through a flute. The positive pressure created by retarding the airflow through pursed lips provides the airways with some stability and with an increased ability to resist surrounding intrapleural pressures. This action works to offset early airway collapse and air trapping during exhalation. In addition, pursed-lip breathing has been shown to slow the patient's ventilatory rate and generates a ventilatory pattern that is more physiologically effective in obstructive pulmonary disease (Fig 1–72).

Polycythemia, Cor Pulmonale

When pulmonary disorders produce chronic hypoxemia, the hormone erythropoietin responds by stimulating the bone marrow to increase red blood cell (RBC) production. RBC production is known as erythropoiesis. An increased level of RBCs is called polycythemia. The *polycythemia* that results from hypoxemia is an adaptive mechanism that increases the oxygen-carrying capacity of the blood.

Cor pulmonale is the term used to denote right ventricular hypertrophy, increased right ventricular work, and ultimately, right ventricular failure. The two major mechanisms involved in producing cor pulmonale in chronic pulmonary disease are (1) the increased viscosity of the blood that is associated with polycythemia and (2) the increased pulmonary vascular resistance caused by hypoxic vasoconstriction.

Increased Viscosity Associated With Polycythemia

Unfortunately, the advantage of the increased oxygen-carrying capacity in polycythemia is offset by the *increased viscosity of the blood* when the hematocrit

experiment, or the possibility of correctly attributing the net effect of the experiment to the role of the intervention. The key is to make sure that the experimental group and the control group are equal at a high confidence level. And a most effective way to achieve this is randomization, i.e., random assignment through the use of a random number table or the technique of systematic sampling. Another approach is called matching, that is, the subjects assigned to the experimental group and those assigned to the control group are paired up to ensure the equality of the two groups on some key variables. The subjects must be stratified before matched assignment. In real terms, perfect matching is impossible because stratification is highly limited in the number of the variables that can be used as criteria for multiple classification. Matching is preferable to randomization, however, when you have very few variables that are considered important and you want to make sure that the subjects are equally assigned on these few variables. On the other hand, although randomization is the precondition for the use of many statistical procedures, it does not provide any guarantee for the equalness of the two groups in any particular study.

Like those factors affecting the external validity of an experimental research, there are some factors that may damage the internal validity of an experimental design (Campbell & Stanley, 1963; Cook & Campbell, 1979). Some of the issues are taken care of by the experimental design itself, yet others need special care in administering the research. Sometimes the problem goes even beyond that due to the limitation of a real research setting, where a classic experimental design has to be compromised as a quasi-experiment. All these may handicap the use of experiments in psychosocial research, though some of the issues will face other forms of research as well.

A special limitation to the use of experimental design in behavioral and social science research is that many psychosocial variables cannot be controlled or manipulated. For instance, to study the consequences of divorce you cannot increase divorce rate by any means since you are bound by research ethics as well as the law not to do this. In such a situation, researchers have to consider non-experimental designs and face a more challenging issue as to how to draw causal conclusions from such studies as cross-sectional surveys.

It should be noted that people tend to refer a social survey only to a non-experimental survey and put it on a par or in contrast with the experimental approach. However, the experimental design should not be considered exclusive to the use of survey methods. In real terms, many experimental studies, especially large-scale social experiments, include the use of survey methods.

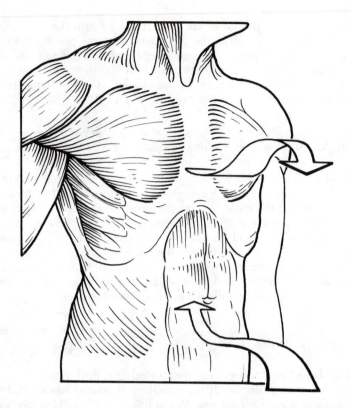

FIG 1–70.
When the accessory muscles of expiration contract, intrapleural pressure increases, the chest moves outward, and bronchial gas flow increases.

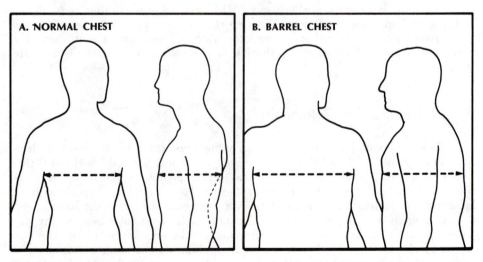

FIG 1–71.
Normally, the ratio of the anteroposterior chest diameter to the lateral chest diameter is about 1:2 **(A).** In patients who have a barrel chest, however, a 1:1 ratio is present **(B).**

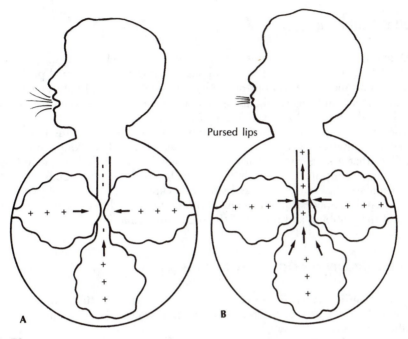

FIG 1–72.
A, schematic illustration of alveoli compression of weakened bronchiole airways during normal expiration in patients with chronic obstructive pulmonary disease (e.g., emphysema). **B,** effects of pursed-lip breathing. The weakened bronchiole airways are kept open by the effects of positive pressure created by pursed lips during expiration.

reaches about 50% to 60%. Because of the increased viscosity of the blood, a greater driving pressure is needed to maintain a given flow. The work of the right ventricle must increase in order to generate the pressure needed to overcome the increased viscosity. This can ultimately lead to right ventricular hypertrophy, or cor pulmonale.

Hypoxic Vasoconstriction of the Pulmonary Vascular System

The decreased arterial oxygen level associated with chronic respiratory disorders causes the smooth muscles of the pulmonary arterioles to contract. The exact mechanism of this phenomenon is unclear. It is known, however, that it is the partial pressure of oxygen in the alveoli ($P_{A_{O_2}}$) and not the partial pressure of arterial oxygen (Pa_{O_2}) that chiefly controls this response.

The effect of hypoxic vasoconstriction is to direct blood away from the hypoxic regions of the lungs and thereby offset the shunt effect. However, when the number of hypoxic regions becomes significant—as during the advanced stages of emphysema—a generalized pulmonary vasoconstriction may develop that may substantially increase pulmonary vascular resistance and the work of the right heart. This in turn can lead to right ventricular hypertrophy and cor pulmonale.

Thus, the cor pulmonale associated with chronic respiratory disorders may develop from the combined effects of polycythemia and pulmonary vasoconstriction. Both of these conditions occur as a result of hypoxemia. Because of the weakness of the right heart in cor pulmonale, venous blood accumulates in the large vessels. In severe cases, this causes the neck veins to become distended, the liver to become enlarged and tender, and the extremities to manifest signs of edema.

Digital Clubbing

Digital clubbing is sometimes noted in patients with chronic respiratory disorders. Clubbing is characterized by a bulbous swelling of the terminal phalanges of the fingers and toes. The contour of the nail becomes rounded both longitudinally and transversely, and this results in an increase in the angle between the surface of the nail and the terminal phalanx (Fig 1–73).

The specific cause of clubbing is unknown. It is believed that the following factors may be causative: (1) circulating vasodilators, such as bradykinin and the prostaglandins, that are released from normal tissues but are not degraduated by the lungs because of intrapulmonary shunting; (2) chronic infection; (3) unspecified toxins; (4) capillary stasis from increased venous backpressure; (4) arterial hypoxia; and (5) local hypoxia. Successful treatment of the underlying disease may result in resolution of the clubbing and return of the digits to normal.

Chest Pain/Decreased Chest Expansion

Chest pain is one of the most common complaints of patients with cardiopulmonary problems. Chest pain can be divided into two categories: pleuritic and nonpleuritic.

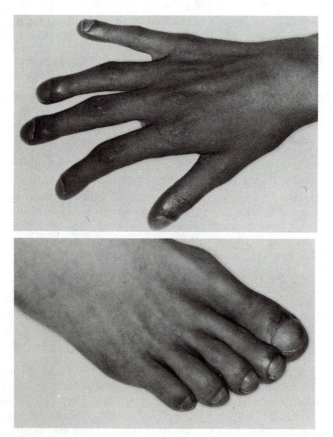

FIG 1–73.
Digital clubbing

Pleuritic Chest Pain

Pleuritic chest pain is usually described as a sudden, sharp, or stabbing pain. The pain generally intensifies during deep inspirations and coughing and diminishes during breath holding or "splinting." The origin of the pain may be the chest wall, muscles, ribs, parietal pleura, diaphragm, mediastinal structures, or intercostal nerves. Since the visceral pleura, which covers the lungs, does not have any sensory nerve supply, pain originating in the parietal region signifies extension of inflammation from the lungs to the contiguous parietal pleura that lines the inner surface of the chest wall. This condition is known as pleurisy (Fig 1–74). When a patient with pleurisy inhales, the lung expands, irritates the inflamed parietal pleura, and causes pain.

Because of the nature of the pleuritic pain, a patient will usually prefer to lie on the side of the pleurisy to allow greater expansion of the uninvolved lung and to help splint the chest on the involved side. Pleuritic chest pain is a characteristic feature of the following respiratory diseases:

- Pneumonia
- Pleural effusion (caused by a pulmonary infection)
- Pneumothorax
- Pulmonary embolism
- Lung cancer
- Pneumonconiosis

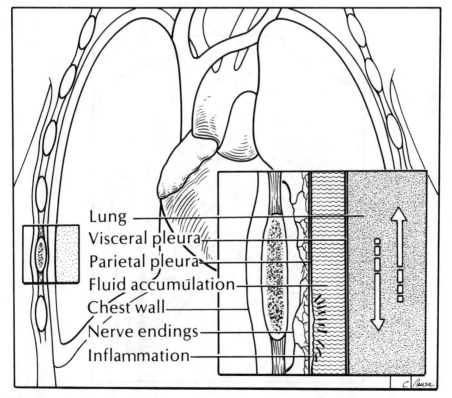

FIG 1–74.
When the parietal pleura is irritated and inflamed, the nerve endings located in the parietal pleura send pain signals to the brain.

- Fungal diseases
- Tuberculosis

Nonpleuritic Chest Pain

Nonpleuritic chest pain is usually described as a constant pain that is located centrally. The pain may also radiate. Nonpleuritic chest pain is associated with the following disorders:

- Myocardial ischemia
- Pericardial inflammation
- Aortic hypertension
- Esophageal inflammation
- Local trauma or inflammation of the chest cage, muscles, bones, or cartilage

Substernal/Intercostal Retractions

Substernal and intercostal retractions may be seen in patients with severe restrictive lung disorders such as pneumonia or adult respiratory distress syndrome. In an effort to overcome the low lung compliance associated with a restrictive lung disorder, the patient must generate a greater-than-normal negative intrapleural pressure during inspiration. This greater negative intrapleural pressure in turn causes the tissues between the ribs and the substernal area to retract inward during inspiration (Fig 1–75). Because the thorax of the newborn is very flexible (due to

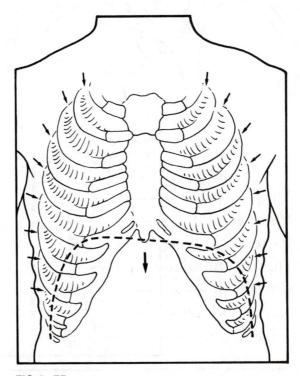

FIG 1–75.
Intercostal retractions of soft tissues during inspiration.

the large amount of cartilage found in the skeletal structure), substernal and inter-costal retractions are commonly seen in the infant with idiopathic respiratory distress syndrome (IRDS).

SELF-ASSESSMENT QUESTIONS

Multiple Choice

1. Which of the following pathologic conditions increases vocal fremitus?
    I. Atelectasis.
    II. Pleural effusion.
    III. Pneumothorax.
    IV. Pneumonia.
        a. III only.
        b. IV only.
        c. II and III only.
        d. I and IV only.
        e. I, III, and IV only.

2. A dull or soft percussion note would likely be heard in which of the following pathologic conditions?
    I. Chronic obstructive pulmonary disease.
    II. Pneumothorax.
    III. Pleural thickening.
    IV. Atelectasis.
        a. I only.
        b. II only.
        c. III only.
        d. II and III only.
        e. III and IV only.

3. Bronchial breath sounds are likely to be heard in which of the following pathologic conditions?
    I. Alveolar consolidation.
    II. Chronic obstructive pulmonary disease.
    III. Atelectasis.
    IV. Fluid accumulation in the tracheobronchial tree.
        a. III only.
        b. IV only.
        c. I and III only.
        d. II and IV only.
        e. I, III, and IV only.

4. In which of the following pathologic conditions is transmission of the whispered voice of a patient through a stethoscope unusually clear?
    I. Chronic obstructive pulmonary disease.
    II. Alveolar consolidation.
    III. Atelectasis.
    IV. Pneumothorax.
        a. I only.
        b. II and III only.
        c. I and IV only.
        d. I, II, and III only.
        e. II, III, and IV only.

5. What is the normal ventilation/perfusion ratio ($\dot{V}/\dot{Q}$ ratio)?
   a. 0.2.
   b. 0.4.
   c. 0.6.
   d. 0.8.
   e. 1.0.

6. If a patient has a $P\bar{E}_{CO_2}$ of 24 mm Hg, a Pa_{CO_2} of 55 mm Hg, and a Pa_{O_2} of 65 mm Hg, approximately what would the V_D/V_T ratio be?
   a. 34%.
   b. 47%.
   c. 56%.
   d. 63%.
   e. 72%.

7. When venous admixture occurs, which of the following occur(s)?
   I. Po_2 of the nonreoxygenated blood increases.
   II. Ca_{O_2} of the reoxygenated blood decreases.
   III. Po_2 of the reoxygenated blood increases.
   IV. Ca_{O_2} of the nonreoxygenated blood decreases.
   a. I only.
   b. IV only.
   c. II and III only.
   d. III and IV only.
   e. I and II only.

8. What percentage is the normal anatomic shunt?
   a. 2–5.
   b. 6–8.
   c. 9–10.
   d. 11–15.
   e. 15–20.

9. When the systemic blood pressure increases, the aortic and carotid sinus barore-ceptors initiate reflexes that cause
   I. Increased heart rate.
   II. Decreased ventilatory rate.
   III. Increased ventilatory rate.
   IV. Decreased heart rate.
   a. I only.
   b. II only.
   c. III only.
   d. II and IV only.
   e. I and III only.

10. What is the average compliance of the lungs and chest wall combined?
    a. 0.05 L/cm H_2O.
    b. 0.1 L/cm H_2O.
    c. 0.2 L/cm H_2O.
    d. 0.3 L/cm H_2O.
    e. 0.4 L/cm H_2O.

11. When lung compliance decreases, the patient's
    I. Ventilatory rate usually decreases.
    II. Tidal volume usually decreases.

   III. Ventilatory rate usually increases.

   IV. Tidal volume usually increases.

      a. I only.

      b. II only.

      c. III only.

      d. II and III only.

      e. I and IV only.

12. What is the normal airway resistance in the tracheobronchial tree?

      a. 0.5–1.0 cm H_2O/L/sec.

      b. 1.0–2.0 cm H_2O/L/sec.

      c. 2.0–3.0 cm H_2O/L/sec.

      d. 3.0–4.0 cm H_2O/L/sec.

      e. 4.0–5.0 cm H_2O/L/sec.

13. In an obstructive lung disorder,

    I. FRC is decreased.

   II. RV is increased.

  III. VC is decreased.

  IV. IRV is increased.

      a. I and III only.

      b. II and III only.

      c. II and IV only.

      d. II, III, and IV only.

      e. I, II, and III only.

14. What is the PEFR in the normal healthy female between 20 and 30 years of age?

      a. 250 L/min.

      b. 350 L/min.

      c. 450 L/min.

      d. 550 L/min.

      e. 650 L/min.

15. Which of the following can be obtained from a flow-volume loop study?

    I. MEFV.

   II. PEFR.

  III. FEVT.

  IV. $FEF_{25\%-75\%}$.

      a. IV only.

      b. I and II only.

      c. II and III only.

      d. I, III, and IV only.

      e. I, II, III, and IV.

16. Bernoulli's principle states that when gas flow through a tube encounters a restriction, the

    I. Velocity of the gas molecules decreases.

   II. Lateral gas pressure decreases.

  III. Velocity of the gas molecules increases.

  IV. Lateral gas pressure increases.

   V. Velocity of the gas molecules remains the same.

      a. II and V only.

      b. II and IV only.

      c. I and IV only.

      d. II and III only.

      e. IV and V only.

17. When arranged for flow ($\dot{V}$), Poiseuille's law states that $\dot{V}$ is
    I. Indirectly related to r^4.
    II. Directly related to P.
    III. Indirectly related to π.
    IV. Directly related to l.
       a. I only.
       b. II only.
       c. II and III only.
       d. III and IV only.
       e. II, III, and IV only.

18. When lactic acidosis is present, the
    I. pH will likely be lower than expected for a particular Pa_{CO_2}.
    II. HCO_3^- will likely be higher than expected for a particular Pa_{CO_2}.
    III. pH will likely be higher than expected for a particular Pa_{CO_2}.
    IV. HCO_3^- will likely be lower than expected for a particular Pa_{CO_2}.
       a. I only.
       b. II only.
       c. III only.
       d. II and III only.
       e. I and IV only.

19. During acute alveolar hyperventilation,
    I. HCO_3^- decreases.
    II. Blood P_{CO_2} increases.
    III. H_2CO_3 decreases.
    IV. $P_{A_{CO_2}}$ increases.
       a. I only.
       b. II only.
       c. III only.
       d. I and III only.
       e. II and IV only.

20. Cardiac output and blood pressure begin to decline when the heart rate increase beyond
       a. 100–125 beats per minute.
       b. 125–150 beats per minute.
       c. 150–175 beats per minute.
       d. 175–200 beats per minute.
       e. 200–250 beats per minute.

21. It is estimated that the cilia move the mucous blanket at an average rate of
       a. 1 cm/min.
       b. 2 cm/min.
       c. 3 cm/min.
       d. 4 cm/min.
       e. 5 cm/min.

22. Which of the following muscles originate from the sternum and from the clavicle?
    I. Scalene muscles.
    II. Sternocleidomastoid muscles.
    III. Pectoralis major muscles.
    IV. Trapezius muscles.
       a. I only.
       b. II only.
       c. IV only.
       d. I and IV only.
       e. II and III only.

23. Which of the following muscles insert into the xyphoid process and into the fifth, sixth, and seventh ribs?
   a. Rectus abdominis muscle.
   b. External oblique muscle.
   c. Internal oblique muscle.
   d. Transversus abdominis muscle.

24. What is the anteroposterior-transverse chest diameter in the normal adult?
   a. 1:05.
   b. 1:1.
   c. 1:2.
   d. 1:3.
   e. 1:4.

25. Which of the following is associated with digital clubbing?
   I. Chronic infection.
   II. Local hypoxia.
   III. Circulating vasodilators.
   IV. Arterial hypoxia.
   a. II only.
   b. IV only.
   c. II and IV only.
   d. II, III, and IV only.
   e. I, II, III, and IV.

26. Which of the following is associated with pleuritic chest pain?
   I. Lung cancer.
   II. Pneumonia.
   III. Myocardial ischemia.
   IV. Tuberculosis.
   a. I only.
   b. II only.
   c. III only.
   d. I and III only.
   e. I, II, and IV only.

True or False

1. Wheezing and rhonchi are typically heard during inspiration.   True ____   False ____

2. When used as accessory muscles of inspiration, the scalene muscles elevate the first and second ribs.   True ____   False ____

3. A decreased partial pressure of oxygen in the alveoli ($P_{A_{O_2}}$) will cause smooth muscle constriction of the pulmonary arterioles.   True ____   False ____

4. The presence of cyanosis is influenced by the temperature of the patient.   True ____   False ____

5. Most of the mucous blanket is produced by the goblet cells.   True ____   False ____

6. Acute changes in the H_2CO_3 level play a much more powerful role in altering the pH status than do acute changes in the HCO_3^- level.   True ____   False ____

7. The blood-brain barrier is relatively impermeable to CO_2 molecules.   True ____   False ____

8. Increased venous pressure and decreased systemic blood pressure are associated with pleural effusions.   True ____   False ____

Data collection methods

The methods of data collection depend on the types of data and where the data will come from. There are two different sources of data, that is, one that is directly collected from the subjects and one that is indirectly available. Indirect data are considered unobtrusive measures since they do not involve the influence of the research process on the subjects being studied.

The first kind of indirect data is that collected, prepared, and often quantified by others, including individual researchers and various public and private organizations. These include various computerized and used data files, published data in aggregated and tabulated forms, business files and reports, and government documents and statistics. The use of such data sources is usually called secondary data analysis. Making use of computerized data collected by other researchers is like joining their teams after the data are collected, cleaned, and analyzed to certain degrees. If the principal investigators permit you to use their data, they will tell you where they are located and how to retrieve them. If you desire to use some large public databases (such as on-line census data) you may need to consult your librarians or statistical experts employed in your computer center. You need to familiarize yourself with the data sets, assess them, adapt to them, and change them to suit your research needs. The advantages and disadvantages of using this kind of data are briefly discussed in chapter three. Basically, you save a lot of time planning, collecting, and cleaning the data; yet, the existing data sets may not provide you with all the information you need. Especially, those public access databases may contain only few core variables that would interest you.

Another important source of the kind of indirect data is compiled or published documentation that gives all sorts of statistics. You can find them in your own library, or you can get them through interlibrary loans. Sometimes you need to contact different agencies and organizations, such as government departments and the chambers of commerce, to request copies of the publications containing the information you need. The statistics give aggregated information beyond the individual, which is frequently used in historical and comparative studies about groups, communities, states, or other forms of human and social entities. You must be aware, however, that such data may have various limitations or reliability and validity problems. There are even more pitfalls in comparative studies due to the differences between social and information reporting systems. Your experience, expertise, as well as good logical reasoning are crucial in making

9. Substernal and intercostal retractions are associated
   with restrictive lung disorders.   True _____   False _____
10. Pursed-lip breathing is commonly used by patients
    with restrictive lung disorders.   True _____   False _____

Clinical Application of the Ideal Alveolar Gas Equation

If a patient is receiving an $F_{I_{O_2}}$ of 55% on a day when the barometric pressure is 745 mm Hg and has a Pa_{CO_2} of 50 mm Hg, what is the patient's calculated PA_{O_2}?

*Answer:*_____

Clinical Application of the Shunt Equation

A 48-year-old woman is on a volume-cycled mechanical ventilator on a day when the barometric pressure is 745 mm Hg. She is receiving intermittent mandatory ventilation of 7 breaths per minute and an $F_{I_{O_2}}$ of .70. The following clinical values are obtained:

Pa_{CO_2}: 46.
Pa_{O_2}: 60 (90% saturated).
$P\bar{v}_{O_2}$: 38 (75% saturated).
Hb: 11 gm/dL.

Based on the above clinical information, how much intrapulmonary shunting does the patient have?

1. PA_{O_2} = _____.
2. Cc_{O_2} = _____.
3. Ca_{O_2} = _____.
4. $C\bar{v}_{O_2}$ = _____.
5. Qs/Q_T = _____.

Matching

Directions: On the line next to the pulmonary function test in column A, match the normal finding for the healthy male between the ages of 20 and 30 years of age in column B. Items in column B may be used once, more than once, or not at all.

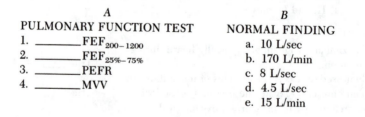

	A PULMONARY FUNCTION TEST		B NORMAL FINDING
1.	_____ $FEF_{200-1200}$	a.	10 L/sec
2.	_____ $FEF_{25\%-75\%}$	b.	170 L/min
3.	_____ PEFR	c.	8 L/sec
4.	_____ MVV	d.	4.5 L/sec
		e.	15 L/min

Answers appear in Appendix XVII.

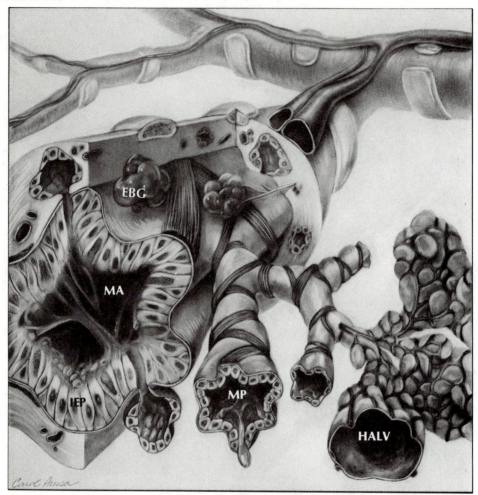

CHRONIC BRONCHITIS

FIG 2–1.
Chronic bronchitis. *EBG* = enlarged bronchial gland; *MA* = mucus accumulation; *IEP* = inflamed epithelium; *MP* = mucus plug; *HALV* = hyperinflated alveoli.

CHRONIC BRONCHITIS

ANATOMIC ALTERATIONS OF THE LUNGS

The conducting airways are the primary structures that undergo anatomic changes in chronic bronchitis. This is particularly true for the peripheral airways. Due to chronic inflammation the bronchial walls are narrowed by vasodilation, congestion, and mucosal edema. Continued bronchial irritation causes the bronchial glands to enlarge and the number of goblet cells to increase, resulting in excessive mucus production. The number of cilia lining the tracheobronchial tree is diminished, and the peripheral bronchi are often partially or totally occluded by inflammation and mucus plugs, which in turn leads to hyperinflated alveoli (Fig 2–1).

To summarize, the following major pathologic or structural changes are associated with chronic bronchitis:

• Chronic inflammation and swelling of the peripheral airways
• Excessive mucus production and accumulation
• Bronchial airway obstruction
• Hyperinflated alveoli

ETIOLOGY

Although the exact cause of chronic bronchitis is not known, the following are thought to be important etiologic factors.

Cigarette Smoking.—Cigarette smoking clearly plays a major etiologic role in chronic bronchitis. Individuals who smoke are much more prone to develop chronic bronchitis than are nonsmokers. Inhaled cigarette smoke contains literally thousands of particles, many of which are irritants that cause bronchial inflammation and destruction of ciliary activity. The excess mucus that accumulates due to decreased ciliary activity increases the patient's vulnerability to secondary bronchial infections, which may further compromise an already inflamed bronchial mucosa.

Atmospheric Pollutants.—Common atmospheric pollutants such as sulfur dioxide, the nitrogen oxides, and ozone are believed to play a significant etiologic role in chronic bronchitis. Prolonged exposure to sulfur dioxide is known to increase airway resistance, and ozone, present in smog, is a well-known respiratory tract irritant. Epidemiologic data reveal an increased morbidity from lung disease in areas of high air pollution.

Infections.—Although the role of infections in causing chronic bronchitis is uncertain, there is evidence that individuals who have repeated respiratory tract infections during childhood are likely to develop chronic bronchitis later in life. Because of the inability of the tracheobronchial tree to clear the excess mucus associated with chronic bronchitis, additional infections compromise the already damaged bronchial tree, and a vicious cycle develops.

OVERVIEW OF THE CARDIOPULMONARY CLINICAL MANIFESTATIONS ASSOCIATED WITH CHRONIC BRONCHITIS*

INCREASED RESPIRATORY RATE
Several pathophysiologic mechanisms operating simultaneously may lead to an increased ventilatory rate. These are (see page 23):

- Stimulation of peripheral chemoreceptors
- Anxiety

PULMONARY FUNCTION STUDIES

EXPIRATORY MANEUVER FINDINGS (see page 38)
- Decreased FVC
- Decreased $FEF_{200-1,200}$
- Decreased $FEF_{25\%-75\%}$
- Decreased FEV_T
- Decreased FEV_1/FVC ratio
- Decreased MVV
- Decreased PEFR
- Decreased $\dot{V}_{max\ 50}$

↓ Flows

LUNG VOLUME AND CAPACITY (see page 47)
- Increased V_T
- Increased RV
- Increased RV/TLC ratio
- Increased FRC
- Increased CV
- Decreased VC
- Decreased IRV
- Decreased ERV

↑ Volumes

INCREASED HEART RATE, CARDIAC OUTPUT, AND BLOOD PRESSURE (see page 57)

*Chronic bronchitis and pulmonary emphysema frequently occur together as a disease complex referred to as chronic obstructive pulmonary disease (COPD). Patients with COPD typically demonstrate clinical manifestations related to both chronic bronchitis and emphysema.

INCREASED ANTEROPOSTERIOR CHEST DIAMETER (BARREL CHEST) (see page 67)

PURSED-LIP BREATHING (see page 67)

USE OF ACCESSORY MUSCLES DURING INSPIRATION (see page 61)

USE OF ACCESSORY MUSCLES DURING EXPIRATION (see page 64)

ARTERIAL BLOOD GASES

EARLY STAGES OF CHRONIC BRONCHITIS
ACUTE ALVEOLAR HYPERVENTILATION WITH HYPOXEMIA (see page 48)

- Pa_{O_2}: decreased
- Pa_{CO_2}: decreased
- HCO_3^-: decreased
- pH: increased

ADVANCED STAGE OF CHRONIC BRONCHITIS
CHRONIC VENTILATORY FAILURE WITH HYPOXEMIA (see page 53)

- Pa_{O_2}: decreased
- Pa_{CO_2}: increased
- HCO_3^-: increased
- pH: normal

CYANOSIS (see page 16)

POLYCYTHEMIA, COR PULMONALE (see page 67)

- Distension of neck veins
- Enlarged and tender liver
- Peripheral edema

CHEST ASSESSMENT FINDINGS (see page 3)

- Decreased tactile and vocal fremitus
- Hyperresonant percussion note
- Diminished breath sounds
- Crackles/rhonchi/wheezing

COUGH AND SPUTUM PRODUCTION (see page 58)

The American Thoracic Society's definition of chronic bronchitis is based on a major clinical manifestation of the disease. The definition states that chronic bronchitis is characterized by a daily, productive cough for at least 3 consecutive months each year for 2 years in a row. Common bacteria found in the bronchial secretions of patients with chronic bronchitis are *Streptococcus pneumoniae* and *Haemophilus influenzae.*

CHEST X-RAY FINDINGS

- Translucency
- Depressed or flattened diaphragm
- Spikelike projections in the bronchogram
- Enlarged heart

There may be no x-ray abnormalities in chronic bronchitis if only the large bronchi are affected. If the more peripheral bronchi are involved, however, there may be substantial air trapping. In the advanced stages of chronic bronchitis, the density of the lungs decreases, and consequently the resistance to x-ray penetration is not as great. This is revealed on x-ray films as areas of translucency or areas that are darker in appearance.

Due to the increased residual volume and functional residual capacity, the diaphragm may be depressed or flattened and is seen in this position on x-ray films (Fig 2–2).

Small spikelike protrusions from the larger bronchi are often seen on bronchograms of persons with chronic bronchitis. It is believed that the spikes result from pooling of the radiopaque medium in the enlarged ducts of the mucus glands. Finally, since venticular heart enlargement and failure often develop as secondary problems during the advanced stages of chronic bronchitis, an enlarged heart may be identified on x-ray films.

INCREASED REID INDEX

Chronic bronchitis can also be diagnosed by the Reid index. The Reid index is the ratio of the bronchial gland thickness to the bronchial wall thickness.

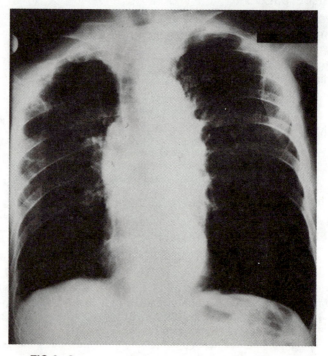

FIG 2–2.
Chest x-ray film of a patient with chronic bronchitis.

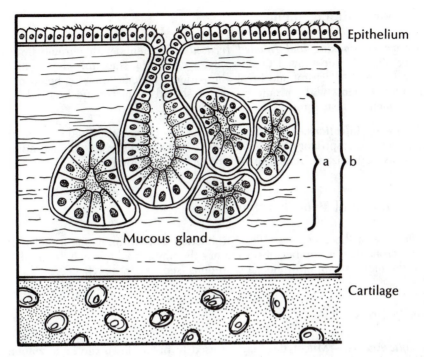

FIG 2–3.
Reid index. **a** represents the size of the mucous gland; **b** represents the size of the lamina propria. When the ratio of the mucous gland and the lamina propria is greater than 0.36, chronic bronchitis is usually present.

Normally this ratio is small; however, when the bronchial mucous glands enlarge, the Reid index becomes larger. If this index is greater than 0.36, chronic bronchitis is generally present (Fig 2–3). This ratio is usually obtained from the average measurements of three to five histologic transverse sections from the main, lobar, or segmental bronchi. Today, the validity of this diagnostic index is questioned.

GENERAL MANAGEMENT OF CHRONIC BRONCHITIS

Patient and Family Education

Both the patient and the patient's family should be given instruction on the patient's disease and its general effects on the body. They should also be instructed in home care therapies, the objectives of these therapies, and how to administer medications. As with emphysema patients, a complete rehabilitation team is sometimes necessary in the management of patients with chronic bronchitis. Such teams include a respiratory therapist, physical therapist, respiratory nurse specialist, occupational therapist, dietitian, social worker, and psychologist. An internist trained in respiratory rehabilitation usually outlines and orchestrates the patient's therapeutic program.

Behavioral Management

Avoidance of Smoking and Inhaled Irritants.—Patients with chronic bronchitis must be strongly encouraged to stop smoking. A "stop-smoking" clinic with techniques designed to disrupt and break the patient's specific smoking behaviors may be helpful. Patients with chronic bronchitis should be instructed to avoid inhaled irritants such as dust, fumes, mist, and toxic gases.

Avoidance of Infections.—Patients with chronic bronchitis should avoid people with contagious respiratory tract infections, especially influenza. Annual immunization against influenza is frequently ordered for these patients.

Mobilization of Bronchial Secretions

Because of the excessive mucus production and accumulation associated with chronic bronchitis, a number of respiratory therapy modalities may be used to enhance the mobilization of bronchial secretions (see Appendix XI).

Medications

Mucolytic Agents.—Mucolytics may be used to break down the large amounts of thick tenacious mucus (see Appendix VI).

Sympathomimetics.—Sympathomimetic drugs are commonly administered to patients with chronic bronchitis to offset bronchial spasms (see Appendix II).

Parasympatholytic Agents.—Parasympatholytic agents are also used to offset bronchial smooth muscle constriction (see Appendix III).

Xanthine Bronchodilators.—Xanthine bronchodilators are used to enhance bronchial smooth muscle relaxation (see Appendix IV).

Expectorants.—Expectorants are often used when water alone is not sufficient to facilitate expectoration (see Appendix VII).

Antibiotics.—Antibiotics are commonly administered to combat or prevent secondary respiratory tract infections (see Appendix VIII).

Positive Inotropic Agents.—When heart failure is present, positive inotropic drugs are commonly administered to increase the cardiac output (see Appendix IX).

Supplemental Oxygen

Because of the hypoxemia associated with chronic bronchitis, supplemental oxygen may be required. The hypoxemia that develops in chronic bronchitis is most commonly caused by the hypoventilation and shuntlike effect associated with the disorder. Hypoxemia caused by a shuntlike effect can generally be corrected by oxygen therapy.

It should be noted, however, that when the patient demonstrates chronic ventilatory failure during the advanced stages of chronic bronchitis, caution must be taken not to eliminate the patient's hypoxic drive to breathe.

SELF-ASSESSMENT QUESTIONS

Multiple Choice

1. In chronic bronchitis
   I. The bronchial walls are narrowed due to vasoconstriction.
   II. The bronchial glands are enlarged.
   III. The number of goblet cells is decreased.
   IV. The number of cilia lining the tracheobronchial tree is increased.
   a. I only.
   b. II only.
   c. III only.
   d. III and IV only.
   e. II, III, and IV only.

2. Which of the following is/are believed to play a major etiologic role in chronic bronchitis?
   I. Ozone.
   II. Nitrous oxide.
   III. Sulfur dioxide.
   IV. Nitrogen oxides.
   a. I only.
   b. II only.
   c. III only.
   d. II and IV only.
   e. I, III, and IV only.

3. Common bacteria found in the tracheobronchial tree of patients with chronic bronchitis is/are
   I. *Staphylococcus.*
   II. *Haemophilus influenzae.*
   III. *Klebsiella.*
   IV. *Streptococcus.*
   a. I only.
   b. II only.
   c. III and IV only.
   d. II and IV only.
   e. I, II, and IV only.

4. When arranged for flow ($\dot{V}$), Poiseuille's law states that $\dot{V}$ is
   I. Indirectly related to P.
   II. Directly related to π.
   III. Indirectly related to l.
   IV. Directly related to r^4.
   a. I and III only.
   b. III only.
   c. II and IV only.
   d. I, II, and III only.
   e. II, III, and IV only.

5. In chronic bronchitis, the patient commonly demonstrates
   I. Increased FVC.
   II. Decreased ERV.
   III. Increased VC.
   IV. Decreased CV.
   a. II only.
   b. III only.

sense out of all the numbers and descriptions.

The second kind of indirect data involves more work in data collection and preparation, but the data collection does not directly deal with human subjects. It only deals with materials or artifacts such as books, journals, magazines, newspapers, and letters, even though the units of analysis could be the authors. Virtually any form of human communication can be the raw material to form the data. Research conducted on this kind of data is called documentary analysis. The technique used to transform such material to statistically manipulable data is called content analysis. It identifies the absence, presence, and frequency of some item(s) in the data being examined. All the research steps we have discussed so far including conceptualization, operationalization, coding and sampling apply to studies using content analysis, though your units of analysis may tend to be some artifacts rather than human subjects. You need, for example, a coding scheme to take the measures and record the data in conducting a content analysis, such as investigating certain advertisements by watching the TV commercials. The traditional way of recording the data in content analysis is to manually put down the counts on a tally sheet for each variable on all its values. For computerized textual documents you can now use some software programs to expedite the work. Maybe someday we will be able to cast away the tally sheets and use the computer with even TV program content analysis (explore this with your computer buddies!).

Despite the convenience (economy), safety (comfort), and stability (durability) that indirect data can provide you, you may need or desire direct data collection for some of your research projects. In real terms, direct data collection is the basic and major form of psychosocial research, which actually produces many indirect data sources for people to use. Compared with content analysis of the artifacts, a methodological issue in direct data collection is the effect of the research procedures on the behavior of the subjects. Many subtle issues may pose a threat to the reliability and validity of the research results. As has been discussed earlier, research design may help to address some of the issues by such means as the modification of the structure of an experiment. The issues will be discussed again in light of the methods and techniques of direct data collection.

When talking about research strategies, particularly data collection methods, you will often read such words as "structured" and "unstructured" from standard methodology texts. These are presented as if they are alternative choices that are equally desirable. It is true that an inquiry without planning and structure may have some utility, especially when pre-structuring a research or data collection

      c. I and III only.

      d. III and IV only.

      e. I, III, and IV only.

6. A trade name of albuterol is
   - I. Proventil.
   - II. Ventolin.
   - III. Vanceril.
   - IV. Brethine.
       - a. I only.
       - b. IV only.
       - c. I and II only.
       - d. III and IV only.
       - e. II, III, and IV only.

7. Chronic bronchitis is generally present when the Reid index is greater than
   - a. 0.03.
   - b. 0.06.
   - c. 0.16.
   - d. 0.26.
   - e. 0.36.

8. The trade name of ipratropium bromide is:
   - a. Theophylline.
   - b. Atropine sulfate.
   - c. Atrovent.
   - d. Guaifenesin.
   - e. Erythromycin.

9. The generic name of Lanoxin is
   - a. Inocor.
   - b. Deslanoside.
   - c. Digitoxin.
   - d. Crystodigin.

10. Which of the following is present during the advanced stages of chronic bronchitis?
    - I. Air trapping.
    - II. Venous admixture.
    - III. Alveolar hyperventilation.
    - IV. Shuntlike effect.
        - a. I and III only.
        - b. II and IV only.
        - c. III and IV only.
        - d. I, II, and III only.
        - e. I, II, and IV only.

Answers appear in Appendix XVII.

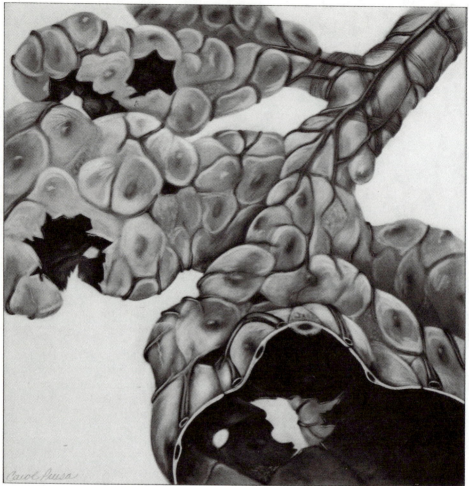

PANLOBULAR EMPHYSEMA

FIG 3–1.
Panlobular emphysema. Abnormal weakening and enlargement of all air spaces distal to the terminal bronchioles.

EMPHYSEMA

ANATOMIC ALTERATIONS OF THE LUNGS

Emphysema is characterized by an abnormal weakening and permanent enlargement of the air spaces distal to the terminal bronchioles and by destruction of the alveolar walls. As these structures enlarge and the alveoli coalesce, many of the adjacent pulmonary capillaries are also affected, and this results in a decreased area for gas exchange. Furthermore, the distal airways, weakened by emphysema, collapse during expiration in response to increased intrapleural pressure. This action traps gas in the distal alveoli. There are two major types of emphysema: panacinar (panlobular) emphysema and centriacinar (centrilobular) emphysema.

In *panlobular emphysema* there is an abnormal weakening and enlargement of all air spaces distal to the terminal bronchioles, including the respiratory bronchioles, alveolar ducts, alveolar sacs, and alveoli. The alveolar-capillary surface area is significantly decreased (Fig 3–1). Panlobular emphysema is commonly found in the lower parts of the lungs and is usually associated with α_1-antitrypsin deficiency.

Centrilobular emphysema primarily involves the respiratory bronchioles in the proximal portion of the acinus. The respiratory bronchiolar walls enlarge, become confluent, and are then destroyed. There is usually a rim of parenchyma that remains relatively unaffected (Fig 3–2). Centrilobular emphysema is the most common form of emphysema and is often associated with chronic bronchitis.

To summarize, the following are the major pathologic or structural changes associated with emphysema:

- Permanent enlargement and deterioration of the air spaces distal to the terminal bronchioles
- Destruction of pulmonary capillaries
- Weakening of the distal airways, primarily the respiratory bronchioles
- Air trapping

ETIOLOGY

Cigarette Smoking.—Although the exact mechanism is unknown, cigarette smoking is thought to be one of the most important etiologic factors in emphysema. Cigarette smoke contains numerous irritants that stimulate mucus production and ultimately impair or destroy ciliary transport. The excess mucus that accumulates as a result of decreased ciliary activity increases the patient's vulnerability to respiratory

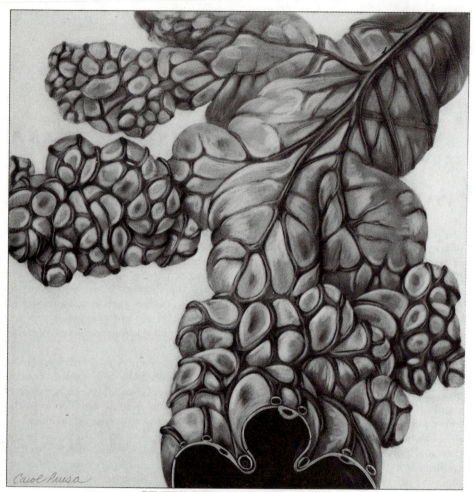

CENTRILOBULAR EMPHYSEMA

FIG 3–2.
Centrilobular emphysema. Abnormal weakening and enlargement of the respiratory bronchioles in the proximal portion of the acinas.

tract infections. Cigarette smoking also causes bronchoconstriction, which in turn increases airway resistance and further impedes tracheobronchial clearance.

α₁-Antitrypsin Deficiency.—It has been noted for many years that panlobular emphysema occurs with unusual frequency in certain families and affects mostly young adults. It is now known that a genetic α_1-antitrypsin deficiency is the key to the high incidence of panlobular emphysema in some families.

α_1-Antitrypsin is a serum glycoprotein that inhibits several proteolytic enzymes. It is synthesized and secreted by the liver. When old white blood cells are destroyed in the lungs, an *elastase* is released that in turn destroys elastic tissue. α_1-Antitrypsin is the enzyme responsible for inactivating the elastase.

The normal level of α_1-antitrypsin is 0.20 to 0.40 gm/100 mL and is genetically referred to as an MM or simply an M phenotype (homozygote). The phenotype associated with the lower serum concentration is ZZ, or simply Z. The heterozygous offspring of parents with the M and Z phenotypes have the phenotype MZ. The MZ phenotype results in an intermediate deficiency of α_1-antitrypsin. The precise role of the intermediate level of α_1-antitrypsin is unclear. It is strongly recommended, however, that these individuals not smoke or work in areas having significant amounts of fumes and dust.

Infections.—There is indirect evidence that repeated respiratory tract infections during childhood may cause permanent airway damage that may eventually develop into chronic obstructive pulmonary disease in adult life.

Inhaled Irritants.—Common atmospheric pollutants such as sulfur dioxide, the nitrogen oxides, and ozone may have an etiologic role in emphysema. Sulfur dioxide is known to increase airway resistance, and ozone, present in smog, is a respiratory tract irritant. Epidemiologic data support the observation that in areas of high air pollution there is increased morbidity from lung disease.

OVERVIEW OF CARDIOPULMONARY CLINICAL MANIFESTATIONS ASSOCIATED WITH EMPHYSEMA*

INCREASED RESPIRATORY RATE
Several pathophysiologic mechanisms operating simultaneously may lead to an increased ventilatory rate. These are (see page 23):

- Stimulation of peripheral chemoreceptors
- Anxiety

PULMONARY FUNCTION STUDIES

EXPIRATORY MANEUVER FINDINGS (see page 38)
- Decreased FVC
- Decreased $FEF_{200-1,200}$
- Decreased $FEF_{25\%-75\%}$
- Decreased FEV_T
- Decreased FEV/FVC ratio
- Decreased MVV
- Decreased PEFR
- Decreased $\dot{V}_{max\ 50}$

LUNG VOLUME AND CAPACITY FINDINGS (see page 47)
- Increased VRT
- Increased RV
- Increased RV/TLC ratio
- Increased FRC
- Increased CV
- Decreased VC
- Decreased IRV
- Decreased ERV

DECREASED DIFFUSION CAPACITY (see page 37)

*Pulmonary emphysema and chronic bronchitis frequently occur together as a disease complex referred to as chronic obstructive pulmonary disease (COPD); therefore patients with COPD typically demonstrate clinical manifestations related to both emphysema and chronic bronchitis.

INCREASED HEART RATE, CARDIAC OUTPUT, AND BLOOD PRESSURE (see page 57)

INCREASED ANTEROPOSTERIOR CHEST DIAMETER (BARREL CHEST) (see page 67)

PURSED-LIP BREATHING (see page 67)

USE OF ACCESSORY MUSCLES DURING INSPIRATION (see page 61)

USE OF ACCESSORY MUSCLES DURING EXPIRATION (see page 64)

ARTERIAL BLOOD GASES

EARLY STAGES OF EMPHYSEMA
ACUTE ALVEOLAR HYPERVENTILATION WITH HYPOXEMIA (see page 48)
- Pa_{O_2}: decreased
- Pa_{CO_2}: decreased
- HCO_3^-: decreased
- pH: increased

ADVANCED STAGES OF EMPHYSEMA
CHRONIC VENTILATORY FAILURE WITH HYPOXEMIA (see page 53)
- Pa_{O_2}: decreased
- Pa_{CO_2}: increased
- HCO_3^-: increased
- pH: normal

CYANOSIS (see page 16)

POLYCYTHEMIA, COR PULMONALE (see page 67)

- Distension of neck veins
- Enlarged and tender liver
- Peripheral edema

DIGITAL CLUBBING (See page 70).

CHEST ASSESSMENT FINDINGS (see page 3)

- Hyperresonant percussion note
- Wheezing
- Diminished breath sounds

CHEST X-RAY FINDINGS

- Translucent
- Depressed or flattened diaphragm
- Enlarged heart

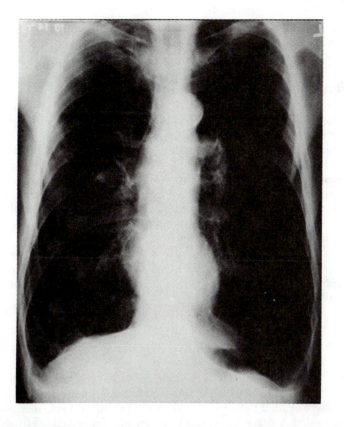

FIG 3–3.
Chest x-ray film of a patient with emphysema. As shown, the heart often appears long and narrow as a result of being drawn downward by the descending diaphragm.

Because of the decreased lung recoil and air trapping that occur in emphysema, the residual volume and functional residual capacity increase. This condition decreases the density of the lungs. Consequently, the resistance to x-ray penetration is not as great. This is revealed on x-ray films as areas of translucency or areas that are darker in appearance. Because of the increased residual volume and functional residual capacity, the diaphragm is depressed or flattened (Fig 3–3). Since ventricular heart enlargement often develops as a secondary problem during the advanced stages of emphysema, an enlarged heart may be seen on x-ray films.

GENERAL MANAGEMENT OF EMPHYSEMA

Patient and Family Education

The patient and the patient's family should be instructed in the type of disease the patient has and how it affects body functions. They should be taught home care therapies, the goals of these therapies, and how to administer medications. For patients with severe emphysema, a pulmonary rehabilitation team is sometimes necessary. Such teams include a respiratory therapist, physical therapist, respiratory nurse specialist, occupational therapist, dietitian, social worker, and psychologist.

An internist trained in respiratory rehabilitation should outline and orchestrate the patient's therapeutic program.

Behavioral Management

Avoidance of Smoking and Inhaled Irritants.—Patients with emphysema must be encouraged to stop smoking. Some patients may need guidance in joining a "stop-smoking" clinic that uses techniques designed to disrupt and break the patient's specific smoking behavior.

The patient should be instructed to avoid inhaled irritants and to avoid occupations that require frequent exposure to dust, fumes, mist, and toxic gases. In some cases, the patient may be encouraged to move away from a highly polluted environment. High-efficiency particulate air filters or electrostatic filters may be useful in eliminating irritating particulate matter from the air.

Avoidance of Infections.—Patients with emphysema should avoid people with contagious respiratory tract infections, particularly influenza. Patients should be immunized annually against influenza.

Proper Nutrition

Because of the dyspnea and resultant air swallowing and also because of the nausea from medications associated with emphysema, many patients lose their appetite and lose weight. Furthermore, when the patients do eat, their stomachs may become distended and further restrict an already depressed and inadequate diaphragm. Such patients may benefit from a high-protein diet administered in small portions six to eight times a day. Supplemental vitamins should be included in such a diet.

Mobilization of Bronchial Secretions

Because of the mucus production and accumulation associated with emphysema (primarily when emphysema appears as a disease complex with chronic bronchitis), a number of respiratory therapy modalities may be used to enhance the mobilization of bronchial secretions (see Appendix XI).

Medications

Sympathomimetics.—Sympathomimetic drugs are frequently administered to patient's with emphysema with accompanying bronchial spasm (see Appendix II). However, these agents are of no benefit for bronchial wheezing produced by airway deterioration and weakening, which is associated with emphysema.

Parasympatholytic Agents.—Parasympatholytic agents are also used to offset bronchial smooth muscle constriction (see Appendix III).

Xanthine Bronchodilators.—Xanthine bronchodilators are used to enhance bronchial smooth muscle relaxation (see Appendix IV).

Expectorants.—Expectorants are often used when water alone is not sufficient to facilitate expectoration (see Appendix VII).

Antibiotics.—Antibiotics are administered to combat or to prevent secondary respiratory tract infections (see Appendix VIII).

Positive Inotropic Agents.—When heart failure is present, positive inotropic drugs are administered to increase cardiac output (see Appendix IX).

Supplemental Oxygen

Because of the hypoxemia associated with emphysema, supplemental oxygen may be required. The hypoxemia that develops in emphysema is most commonly caused by the hypoventilation and shuntlike effect associated with the disorder. Hypoxemia caused by a shuntlike effect can generally be corrected by oxygen therapy.

It should be noted, however, that when the patient demonstrates chronic ventilatory failure during the advanced stages of emphysema, caution must be taken not to eliminate the patient's hypoxic drive.

SELF-ASSESSMENT QUESTIONS

Multiple Choice

1. The lowest concentration of α_1-antitrypsin is genetically termed
    a. MM phenotype.
    b. MZ phenotype.
    c. ZZ phenotype.
    d. M phenotype.
    e. ZM phenotype.
2. What is the normal level of α_1-antitrypsin?
    a. 0.20–0.40 gm/100 mL.
    b. 0.60–0.80 gm/100 mL.
    c. 0.80–1.00 gm/100 mL.
    d. 1.00–1.20 gm/100 mL.
    e. 2.00–3.00 gm/100 mL.
3. The diffusion capacity of patients with emphysema is
    a. Increased.
    b. Decreased.
    c. Not affected.
4. The chest wall has a natural tendency to
    a. Recoil inward.
    b. Expand outward.
    c. Remain stable.
    d. Recoil inward during expiration.
5. Which accessory muscle of inspiration elevates the first and second ribs?
    a. Scalene muscle.
    b. Sternocleidomastoid muscle.
    c. Internal oblique muscle.
    d. Pectoralis major muscle.
    e. External oblique muscle.

procedure is premature, impractical, or impossible. However, you should understand the difference between unstructured activities and structured inquiry. In a sense, the structure of scientific inquiry is what research methodology is all about, although the whole process of inquiry could be regarded as proceeding from unstructured to semi-structured, and eventually to a structured product. You should plan ahead and give all your activities a structure as much as you can to facilitate the conduct of your research.

Direct data collection may be a process of simple observation that includes watching and listening. Although possible, psychosocial research seldom uses human sensory functions of touching, smelling, or tasting as a major means of data collection. Observation literally means noting and recording, and data are formed in this two-fold process. Nevertheless, data collection can also be a process of questioning, and the answers can be observed by the researcher, or directly recorded by the respondent himself.

Observation has different modes that can be categorized from different angles. Based on the different positions of the researcher, i.e., whether or not he gets involved or takes part in the activity of the group being observed, observation is usually divided into participant observation and nonparticipant observation. Participation or nonparticipation is a relative matter, however. The degree of the researcher's involvement may differ from project to project, and also vary from time to time in a same project. The decision should be made based on the need for obtaining particular kinds of information that demand various degrees of involvement of the observer.

An observation, on the other hand, may be announced or not announced to the group being observed, depending on the researcher's consideration of such consequences as the impact of the presence of the observer (called "interviewer effect") and the ethical responsibility to those being observed. These issues tend to be intensified in the situation of a participant observation.

Observation may take place very naturally, or may be conducted in arranged settings. For the researcher, this is a matter of structure, which we have already discussed. For those being observed, the difference is whether they are acting on their own or under the researcher's directions. Researchers from academic disciplines may introduce some intervention into their research, such as the experimental design. Other than that, they seldom would tell the subjects how they should act. Researchers from practicing professions such as social work and psychotherapy, in contrast, often tell the subjects the entire action plan. They would observe the differences in the clients' way of following the instructions

6. The chest x-ray film of a patient with emphysema is
   I. Opaque.
   II. Whiter in appearance.
   III. More translucent.
   IV. Darker in appearance.
     a. I only.
     b. II only.
     c. I and III only.
     d. II and III only.
     e. III and IV only.

7. During the early stages of emphysema, the patient's Pa_{O_2} decreases because of a progressive
   I. Decrease in the patient's residual volume.
   II. Increase in the patient's functional residual capacity.
   III. Decrease in the patient's ventilation-perfusion ratio.
   IV. Increase in the patient's ventilation-perfusion ratio.
     a. I and II only.
     b. II and III only.
     c. III and IV only.
     d. I and III only.
     e. II and IV only.

8. When arranged for flow ($\dot{V}$), Poiseuille's law states that $\dot{V}$ is
   I. Directly related to r^4.
   II. Indirectly related to π.
   III. Directly related to l.
   IV. Indirectly related to n.
     a. I and II only.
     b. I and IV only.
     c. III and IV only.
     d. II and III only.
     e. II, III, and IV only.

9. Cyanosis is commonly observed when blood hemoglobin is reduced by:
     a. 3 gm/dL.
     b. 5 gm/dL.
     c. 7 gm/dL.
     d. 10 gm/dL.
     e. 15 gm/dL.

10. Which of the following are associated with polycythemia?
    I. Decreased blood viscosity.
    II. Erythropoiesis.
    III. Hypoxemia.
    IV. Cor pulmonale.
      a. I and II only.
      b. II and IV only.
      c. I, III, and IV only.
      d. II, III, and IV only.
      e. I, II, III, and IV.

True or False

1. Panlobular emphysema is the type of emphysema that creates an abnormal enlargement of all structures distal to the terminal bronchioles.   True _____   False _____

2. α_1-Antitrypsin is the enzyme responsible for activating elastase. True _____ False _____

3. α_1-Antitrypsin deficiency is associated with centrilobular emphysema. True _____ False _____

4. You would expect the following abnormal lung volume and capacity findings in patients with emphysema:
   a. Increased residual volume. True _____ False _____
   b. Decreased functional residual capacity. True _____ False _____
   c. Increased expiratory reserve volume. True _____ False _____
   d. Increased inspiratory reserve volume. True _____ False _____

5. You would expect the following abnormal expiratory maneuver findings in patients with emphysema:
   a. Decreased forced expiratory flow, 25%–75%. True _____ False _____
   b. Increased maximum voluntary ventilation. True _____ False _____

6. A patient during the late stage of emphysema commonly has the following arterial blood gas values:
   a. Decreased Pa_{CO_2}. True _____ False _____
   b. A pH and HCO_3^- reading that indicate the presence of lactic acid accumulation. True _____ False _____

Fill in the Blank

1. The single most important etiologic factor in emphysema is thought to be
   _____.

2. The limitation of the flow rate that occurs during approximately the last 70% of a forced vital capacity maneuver is due to _____ compression of the airway walls.

3. As the airway pressure decreases from the alveolus to the atmosphere during a forced expiratory maneuver, there eventually comes a point at which the transpulmonary pressure is zero. This is known as the _____.

Answers appear in Appendix XVII.

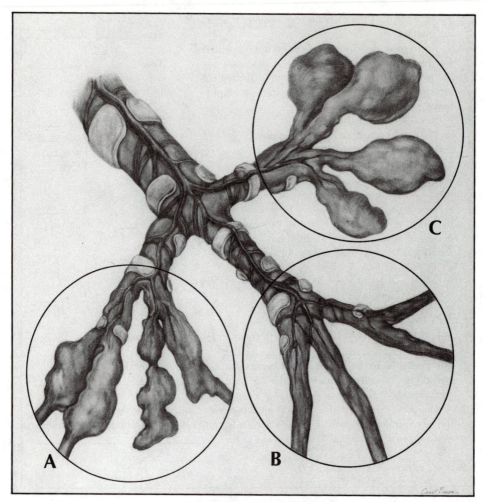

BRONCHIECTASIS

FIG 4–1.
Bronchiectasis. **A,** varicose bronchiectasis. **B,** cylindrical bronchiectasis. **C,** saccular bronchiectasis.

BRONCHIECTASIS

ANATOMIC ALTERATIONS OF THE LUNGS

Bronchiectasis is characterized by chronic dilatation and distortion of one or more bronchi due to extensive inflammation and destruction of the bronchial wall cartilage, blood vessels, elastic tissue, and smooth muscle components. Either or both lungs may be involved. The smaller bronchi, with less supporting cartilage, are predominantly affected.

Because of bronchial wall deterioration, the mucociliary clearing mechanism is impaired, and this results in the accumulation of copious amounts of bronchial secretions that become foul-smelling due to secondary infections. The small bronchi and bronchioles distal to the affected areas become partially—or totally—obstructed with secretions. This condition leads into either one or both of the following anatomic alterations: (1) hyperinflation of the alveoli as a result of expiratory check-valve obstruction or (2) atelectasis and parenchymal fibrosis as a result of complete bronchial obstruction.

Three forms—or anatomic varieties—of bronchiectasis have been described: (1) *varicose (fusiform)*, (2) *cylindrical (tubular)*, and (3) *saccular (cystic)*.

Varicose Bronchiectasis

The bronchi are dilated and constricted in an irregular fashion similar to varicose veins, ultimately resulting in a distorted, bulbous shape (Fig 4–1,A).

Cylindrical Bronchiectasis

The bronchi are dilated and have regular outlines similar to a tube. The dilated bronchi fail to taper for six to ten generations and then end squarely because of mucus obstruction (Fig 4–1,B).

Saccular Bronchiectasis Causes greatest damage

The bronchi progressively increase in diameter until they end in large, cystlike sacs in the lung parenchyma. This form of bronchiectasis causes the greatest damage to the tracheobronchial tree. The bronchial walls become composed of fibrous tissue alone—cartilage, the elastic tissue, and smooth muscle are all absent (Fig 4–1,C).

Today these classifications are no longer considered to be meaningful and are largely abandoned. Bronchiectasis is commonly limited to a lobe or a segment and is frequently found in the left lower lobe.

To summarize, following are the major pathologic or structural changes found in bronchiectasis:

- Chronic dilatation and distortion of bronchial airways
- Excessive production of copious amounts of foul-smelling sputum
- Hyperinflated alveoli
- Atelectasis and parenchymal fibrosis

ETIOLOGY

The etiology of bronchiectasis is not always clear, but there is some evidence indicating that the disease may be either acquired or congenital.

Acquired Bronchiectasis

Pulmonary Infection.—Bronchiectasis is commonly seen in individuals who have repeated and prolonged episodes of respiratory tract infections. Children who have frequent bouts of bronchopneumonia—due to the respiratory complications of measles, chickenpox, pertussis, or influenza, for example—often acquire some form of bronchiectasis later in life.

Bronchial Obstruction.—Bronchial obstruction caused by tumor masses, enlarged hilar lymph nodes, or aspirated foreign bodies may result in bronchiectasis. It is felt that these conditions impair the mucociliary clearing mechanism and this impairment, in turn, favors the development of necrotizing bacterial infections.

Pulmonary Tuberculosis.—Because of the inflammatory process and bronchial wall destruction associated with pulmonary tuberculosis, bronchiectasis is a common secondary complication of this disease.

Congenital Bronchiectasis

Kartagener's Syndrome.—Kartagener's syndrome is a triad consisting of bronchiectasis, dextrocardia (having the heart on the right side of the body), and paranasal sinusitis. Kartagener's syndrome accounts for as much as 20% of all congenital bronchiectasis.

Hypogammaglobulinemia.—Bronchiectasis is commonly seen in individuals who have an inadequate regional or systemic defense mechanism because of an inherited immune deficiency disorder. These individuals have a high predisposition for recurrent episodes of respiratory infections.

Cystic Fibrosis.—Because of impairment of the mucociliary clearing mechanism and the abundance of stagnant, thick mucus associated with cystic fibrosis, bronchial obstruction due to mucus plugging and bronchial infections frequently results. The necrotizing inflammations that develop under these conditions often lead to secondary bronchiectasis.

OVERVIEW OF THE CARDIOPULMONARY CLINICAL MANIFESTATIONS THAT MAY BE ASSOCIATED WITH BRONCHIECTASIS

Depending upon the amount of bronchial secretions and the degree of bronchial deterioration associated with bronchiectasis in its advanced stages, the disease may create either an obstructive or a restrictive lung disorder—or a combination of both. If the majority of the bronchial airways are only partially obstructed, the bronchiectasis will manifest itself primarily as an obstructive lung disorder. If, on the other hand, the majority of the bronchial airways are completely obstructed, the distal alveoli will collapse, and the bronchiectasis will manifest itself primarily as a restrictive disorder. Finally, it should be emphasized that if the disease is limited to a relatively small portion of the lungs—as it often is—the patient may not have any of the following clinical manifestations.

INCREASED RESPIRATORY RATE

Several pathophysiologic mechanisms operating simultaneously may lead to an increased ventilatory rate. These are (see page 23):

- Stimulation of peripheral chemoreceptors
- Decreased Lung Compliance/Increased Work Of Breathing Relationship
- Anxiety

PULMONARY FUNCTION STUDIES

WHEN PRIMARILY OBSTRUCTIVE IN NATURE
EXPIRATORY MANEUVER FINDINGS (see page 38)
- Decreased FVC
- Decreased $FEF_{200-1,200}$
- Decreased $FEF_{25\%-75\%}$
- Decreased FEV_T
- Decreased FEV_1/FVC ratio
- Decreased MVV
- Decreased PEFR
- Decreased $\dot{V}_{max\ 50}$

LUNG VOLUME AND CAPACITY FINDINGS (see page 47)
- Increased V_T
- Increased RV
- Increased RV/TLC ratio
- Increased FRC
- Decreased CV
- Decreased VC
- Decreased IRV
- Decreased ERV

LUNG VOLUME AND CAPACITY FINDINGS (see page 37)
WHEN PRIMARILY RESTRICTIVE IN NATURE

- Decreased VC
- Decreased RV
- Decreased FRC

- Decreased TLC
- Decreased VT

INCREASED HEART RATE, CARDIAC OUTPUT, BLOOD PRESSURE (see page 57)

INCREASED ANTEROPOSTERIOR CHEST DIAMETER (BARREL CHEST) (see page 67)

PURSED-LIP BREATHING (see page 67)

USE OF ACCESSORY MUSCLES DURING INSPIRATION (see page 61)

USE OF ACCESSORY MUSCLES DURING EXHALATION (see page 64)

ARTERIAL BLOOD GASES

EARLY STAGES OF BRONCHIECTASIS
ACUTE ALVEOLAR HYPERVENTILATION WITH HYPOXEMIA (see page 48)
- Pa_{O_2}: decreased
- Pa_{CO_2}: decreased
- HCO_3^-: decreased
- pH: increased

ADVANCED STAGES OF BRONCHIECTASIS
CHRONIC VENTILATORY FAILURE WITH HYPOXEMIA (see page 53)
- Pa_{O_2}: decreased
- Pa_{CO_2}: increased
- HCO_3^-: increased
- pH: normal

CYANOSIS (see page 16)

POLYCYTHEMIA/COR PULMONALE (see page 67)

- Distension of neck veins
- Enlarged and tender liver
- Peripheral edema

DIGITAL CLUBBING (see page 70)

CHEST ASSESSMENT FINDINGS

PRIMARILY OBSTRUCTIVE IN NATURE (see page 3)
- Decreased Tactile and Vocal Fremitus
- Hyperresonant Percussion Note
- Diminished Breath Sounds
- Crackles/Rhonchi/Wheezing

PRIMARILY RESTRICTIVE IN NATURE (see page 3)
- Increased Tactile and Vocal Fremitus
- Bronchial Breath Sounds
- Dull Percussion Notes
- Whispered Pectoriloquy

COUGH, SPUTUM PRODUCTION, AND HEMOPTYSIS (see page 58)

A chronic cough with the production of large quantities of foul-smelling sputum is a hallmark of bronchiectasis. A 24-hour collection of sputum is usually copious and tends to settle into several different layers. Streaks of blood are frequently found in the sputum, presumably originating from necrosis of the bronchial walls and bronchial blood vessels. Frank hemoptysis may also occur from time to time. Because of the excessive bronchial secretions, secondary bacterial infections are frequent. *Haemophilus influenzae* and *Streptococcus* are commonly cultured from the sputum of patients with bronchiectasis.

The productive cough in bronchiectasis is triggered by the large amount of secretions that fill the tracheobronchial tree. The stagnant secretions stimulate the subepithelial mechanoreceptors, which in turn produce a vagal reflex that triggers a cough. Although the subepithelial mechanoreceptors are found in the trachea, bronchi, and bronchioles, they are predominantly located in the upper airways.

CHEST X-RAY FINDINGS

- Bronchography (positive finding)
- Translucencies
- Depressed or flattened diaphragm
- Increased opacity

Bronchography is commonly performed on patients with bronchiectasis. It is the best method of diagnosing bronchiectiasis and delineating the extent and type of tracheobronchial involvement. This procedure entails the injection of an opaque contrast material into the lungs.

In cylindrical bronchiectasis, the bronchogram commonly shows dilated, cylinder-shaped bronchioles (Fig 4–2). There may be increased bronchial markings and adjacent emphysema.

In saccular bronchiectasis, the bronchogram shows large, saclike structures; fibrotic markings; associated atelectasis; and adjacent emphysema.

In varicose bronchiectasis, the bronchogram may show bronchi that are dilated and constricted in an irregular fashion and terminate in a distorted, bulbous shape.

During the advanced stages of bronchiectasis, the alveoli may often become hyperinflated and cause the residual volume and functional residual capacity to increase. On x-ray films this appears as areas that are translucent or darker in appearance. In addition, the diaphragm may be depressed or flattened. Because atelectasis develops in some forms of bronchiectasis, an increased opacity may appear on the x-ray film.

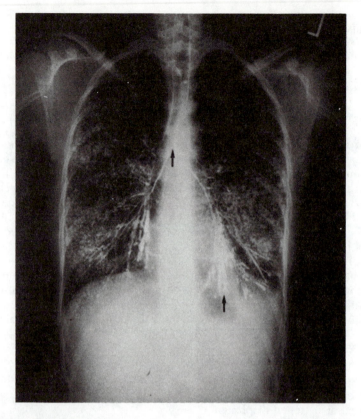

FIG 4–2.
Bronchogram obtained using contrast medium in a patient with a history of bronchiectasis. *Arrows* indicate the carina and the bronchi leading to the posterior basilar segment of the left lower lobe. (From Rau JL Jr, Pearce DJ: *Understanding Chest Radiographs.* Denver, Multi-Media Publishing Inc, 1984. Used by permission.)

GENERAL MANAGEMENT OF BRONCHIECTASIS

Mobilization of Bronchial Secretions

Because of the excessive mucus production and accumulation associated with bronchiectasis, a number of respiratory therapy modalities may be used to enhance the mobilization of bronchial secretions (see Appendix XI).

Medications

Mucolytic Agents.—Mucomyst may be used to break down the large amounts of thick tenacious mucus (see Appendix VI).

Sympathomimetics.—Sympathomimetic drugs are commonly administered to patients with bronchiectasis to offset bronchial spasms (see Appendix II).

Parasympatholytic Agents.—Parasympatholytic agents are also used to offset bronchial smooth muscle constriction (see Appendix III).

Xanthine Bronchodilators.—Xanthine bronchodilators are used to enhance bronchial smooth muscle relaxation (see Appendix IV).

Expectorants.—Expectorants are often used when water alone is not sufficient to facilitate expectoration (see Appendix VII).

Antibiotics.—Antibiotics are administered to combat or to prevent secondary respiratory tract infections (see Appendix VIII).

Positive Inotropic Agents.—When heart failure is present, positive inotropic drugs are administered to increase cardiac output (see Appendix IX).

Supplemental Oxygen

Because of the hypoxemia associated with bronchiectasis, supplemental oxygen may be required. The hypoxemia that develops in bronchiectasis is most commonly caused by the hypoventilation and shuntlike effect associated with the disorder. Hypoxemia caused by a shuntlike effect can generally be corrected by oxygen therapy.

It should be noted, however, that when the patient demonstrates chronic ventilatory failure during the advanced stages of bronchiectasis, caution must be taken not to eliminate the patient's hypoxic drive to breathe.

SELF-ASSESSMENT QUESTIONS

Multiple Choice

1. In which of the following forms of bronchiectasis are the bronchi dilated and constricted in an irregular fashion?
   I. Fusiform.
   II. Saccular.
   III. Varicose.
   IV. Cylindrical.
   a. I only.
   b. II only.
   c. III only.
   d. II and IV only.
   e. I and III only.
2. Which of the following are common causes of acquired bronchiectasis?
   I. Hypogammaglobulinemia.
   II. Pulmonary tuberculosis.
   III. Kartagener's syndrome.
   IV. Cystic fibrosis.
   a. I only.
   b. II only.
   c. III only.
   d. III and IV only.
   e. I, III, and IV only.
3. In the primarily obstructive form of bronchiectasis, the patient commonly demonstrates
   I. Decreased FRC.
   II. Increased $FEF_{25\%-75\%}$.
   III. Decreased PEFR.

and producing the activity outcomes. For these researchers, this is an efficient way of gathering information to serve the purpose of practice, which is buttressed by theoretical traditions such as the psychoanalytic school. For the purpose of research, however, it is not easy to justify why we should spend more time on producing the projections than on gathering the real facts (if possible at all). After all, there does not seem to be enough evidence to show a high correlation between the subjects' way of following the researcher's instructions and the way they live their real lives.

In many cases, simple observation cannot provide sufficient information for research. In other words, social science research often entails the researcher's interaction with the subjects in the form of asking questions to solicit information, in addition to other forms of observation. When the question-answer strategy is used, the research subjects are called respondents. Questions may be verbally asked, or be written and read. The former can be conducted face-to-face or by phone, and the latter can be delivered in person or by mail. In a situation of answering questions in front of a data collector, the observation is announced and the "interviewer effect" should be noted. Here the skills and attitudes of the interviewer are extremely important.

The conversation between the data collector and the respondent, consisting mainly of questions and answers around certain research topics, is called an interview. The data collector, called the interviewer, has the major function of asking the respondent (the interviewee) questions and recording the answers, though sometimes she is also supposed to note and record things observed during the conversation. Note the questions asked of your respondents are usually not the same as your research questions, i.e., the questions you ask of yourself in conducting the research. According to the extent the interview is structured, the interviewer may only have an outline about the interview or a list of questions to be phrased. Or she may have to follow a carefully designed schedule prescribing the exact wording of the questions as well as the procedures to ask for and record the answers. A formal interview instrument, usually a well structured schedule, is called a questionnaire. A questionnaire is a major product of operationalization and research design. The interviewer uses the questionnaire to ask the prepared questions as well as record the answers. Questionnaire interviews are very common in behavioral and social science research, which are especially suited to the study of certain populations (e.g., the elderly), and in some special research situations (e.g., interviewing by telephone).

For some other respondents or for the same respondents in some other

IV. Increased $\dot{V}_{max\ 50}$.
    a. I only.
    b. III only.
    c. I and III only.
    d. II and IV only.
    e. III, and IV only.

4. When arranged for pressure (P), Poiseuille's law states that P is
    I. Directly related to r^4.
    II. Indirectly related to L.
    III. Directly related to $\dot{V}$.
    IV. Indirectly related to n.
      a. I only.
      b. III only.
      c. IV only.
      d. I and II only.
      e. II and IV only.

5. Which of the following are used as accessory muscles of inspiration?
    I. Trapezius muscles.
    II. Transversus abdominis muscle.
    III. Scalene muscle.
    IV. Internal oblique muscle.
      a. I only.
      b. II only.
      c. IV only.
      d. I and III only.
      e. II and IV only.

6. Airway resistance equals
    a. Pressure change divided by flow.
    b. Flow multiplied by pressure change.
    c. Pressure change plus flow.
    d. Flow divided by pressure change.
    e. Pressure change minus flow change.

7. Which of the following is felt to be the best method of diagnosing bronchiectasis?
    a. Chest x-ray.
    b. Pulmonary function study.
    c. Arterial blood gas analysis.
    d. Bronchography.
    e. Ventilation-perfusion lung scan.

8. A trade name of terbutaline is
    I. Brethine.
    II. Albuterol.
    III. Bricanyl.
    IV. Ventolin.
      a. I only.
      b. II only.
      c. III only.
      d. I and III only.
      e. II and IV only.

9. Which of the following is/are commonly cultured in the sputum of patients with bronchiectasis?
    I. *Staphylococcus*.
    II. Klebsiella.
    III. Streptococcus.

    IV. Haemophilus influenzae.
  a. I only.
  b. II only.
  c. III only.
  d. I and III only.
  e. III and IV only.
10. The generic name of Mucomyst is
  a. Triamcinolone acetonide.
  b. *N*-Acetylcystine.
  c. Beclomethasone.
  d. Cromolyn sodium.
  e. Dexamethasone.

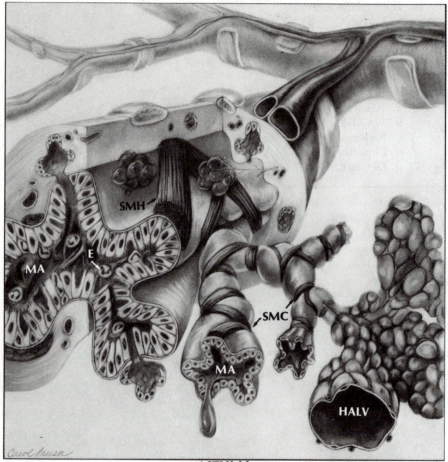

ASTHMA

FIG 5–1.
Asthma. *SMH* = smooth muscle hypertrophy; *MA* = mucus accumulation; *E* = eosinophils; *SMC* = smooth muscle constriction; *HALV* = hyperinflated alveoli.

ASTHMA

ANATOMIC ALTERATIONS OF THE LUNGS

During an asthma attack, the smooth muscles surrounding the small airways of the lungs constrict in response to a particular stimulus. In time the smooth muscle layers hypertrophy and may increase to three times their normal size. There is a proliferation of goblet cells, and the bronchial mucous glands enlarge. The airways become filled with thick, tenacious mucus, and extensive mucus plugging may develop. The bronchial mucosa is edematous and infiltrated with eosinophils. The cilia are damaged, and the basement membrane of the mucosa is thicker than normal. As a result of smooth muscle constriction, bronchial mucosal edema, and hypersecretions, air trapping and alveolar hyperinflation develop. A remarkable feature of bronchial asthma is that the anatomic alterations that occur during an asthmatic attack are completely absent between the asthmatic episodes (Fig 5–1).

To summarize, the major pathologic or structural changes observed during an asthmatic episode are as follows:

- Smooth muscle constriction of bronchial airways
- Excessive production of thick, tenacious tracheobronchial secretions
- Hyperinflation of alveoli

ETIOLOGY

Asthma is divided into two kinds according to the precipitating factors: *extrinsic asthma*, or asthma caused by external or environmental agents, and *intrinsic asthma*, or asthma that occurs in the absence or lack of evidence of an antigen-antibody reaction. While some authorities believe that the distinction between these two terms is of minimal clinical value, the terms are nevertheless widely used.

Extrinsic Asthma (Allergic or Atopic Asthma)

When an asthmatic episode can be clearly associated with exposure to a specific antigenic agent such as pollen, house dust, or feathers, the asthma is referred to as extrinsic. Individuals with extrinsic asthma are said to have an allergic or atopic disorder, which means that the individual demonstrates some type of hypersensitivity to common environmental allergens. Such individuals develop a wheal and flare reaction to a variety of skin allergens. Extrinsic asthma is family related and usually appears in children and in adults under the age of 30 years. It often disappears after puberty.

Because extrinsic asthma is associated with an antigen-antibody–induced bronchospasm, an immunologic mechanism plays an important role. Like other organs,
the lungs are protected against infection by certain immunologic mechanisms. Under normal circumstances, these mechanisms function without any clinical evidence
of their activity. In patients susceptible to extrinsic or allergic asthma, however, it
is the immune response itself that actually creates the disease.

The Immunologic Mechanism

1. When a susceptible individual is exposed to a certain antigen, lymphoid tissue cells form specific IgE (reaginic) antibodies. The IgE antibodies attach themselves to the surface of mast cells in the bronchial walls (Fig 5–2,A).

2. Continued exposure to the same antigen creates an antigen-antibody reaction on the surface of the mast cell, which in turn causes the mast cell to degranu-
late and release chemical mediators such as histamine, slow-reacting substance of
anaphylaxis (SRS-A), eosinophil chemotactic factor of anaphylaxis (ECF-A), and
bradykinin (Fig 5–2,B).

3. The release of these chemical mediators decreases the intracellular levels of
cyclic adenosine monophosphate (cAMP) in the smooth muscles of the bronchi and
causes bronchoconstriction. Moreover, these chemical mediators alter the permeability of capillaries, which results in the dilation of blood vessels and tissue edema
(Fig 5–2,C).

4. This antigen-antibody reaction is thought to trigger an asthmatic episode in
individuals having extrinsic asthma. Furthermore, the production of IgE antibodies
may be 20 times greater than normal in some asthmatic patients. (The normal IgE
antibody level in the serum is about 200 ng/mL).

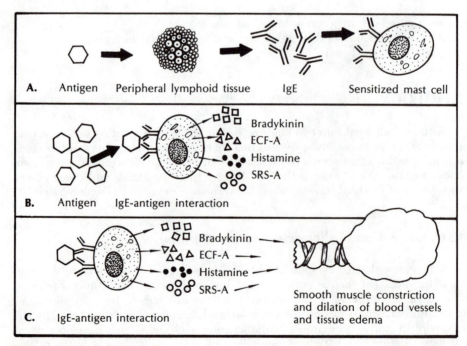

A.   Antigen   Peripheral lymphoid tissue   IgE   Sensitized mast cell

B.   Antigen   IgE-antigen interaction   Bradykinin ECF-A Histamine SRS-A

C.   IgE-antigen interaction   Bradykinin ECF-A Histamine SRS-A   Smooth muscle constriction
and dilation of blood vessels
and tissue edema

FIG 5–2.
The immunologic mechanism.

5. Individuals with extrinsic asthma may demonstrate either a type I or a type III allergic response. The type I response is an immediate allergic reaction that is evoked by the antigen-antibody reaction just described. In a type III reaction the invading antigen chemically combines with another precipitating immunoglobulin, usually of the IgE class, and delays the allergic response for 6 to 8 hours following exposure.

Intrinsic Asthma (Nonallergic or Nonatopic Asthma)

When an asthmatic episode cannot be associated with exposure to a specific external or environmental agent, it is referred to as intrinsic. The etiologic factors responsible for intrinsic asthma are elusive. Individuals with intrinsic asthma are not hypersensitive or atopic to environmental antigens and have a normal serum IgE level. Intrinsic asthma can be triggered by (1) infections, (2) cold air, (3) vapor, (4) industrial or occupational exposure, (5) chemical irritants or fumes, (6) dust and air pollutants, (7) tobacco smoke, (8) drugs (particularly aspirin), (9) emotional stress, and (10) exercise (Fig 5–3).

The onset of intrinsic asthma usually occurs after the age of 35 years, and there is typically no family history of asthma. Chronic bronchitis is a frequent complication, as are bacterial and viral infections.

The β_2-Blockade Theory of Intrinsic Asthma

It has been suggested that a partial β_2-blockade could account for the occurrence of asthma in some individuals. When the β_2-receptors of the autonomic system are blocked, the cAMP level decreases, the cyclic guanosine monophosphate (cGMP) level increases, and the bronchial smooth muscles constrict.

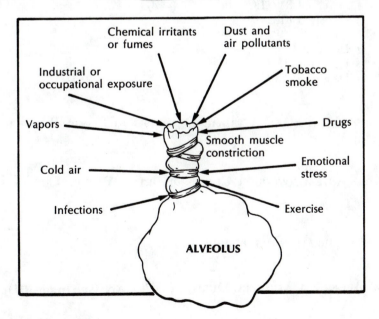

FIG 5–3.
Intrinsic factors triggering asthma.

OVERVIEW OF THE CARDIOPULMONARY CLINICAL MANIFESTATIONS ASSOCIATED WITH AN ASTHMATIC EPISODE

INCREASED RESPIRATORY RATE

Several pathophysiologic mechanisms operating simultaneously may lead to an increased ventilatory rate. These are (see page 23):

- Stimulation of peripheral chemoreceptors
- Decreased lung compliance/increased work of breathing relationship
- Anxiety

PULMONARY FUNCTION STUDIES

EXPIRATORY MANEUVER FINDINGS (see page 38)
- Decreased FVC
- Decreased $FEF_{200-1,200}$ *↓ flows*
- Decreased $FEF_{25\%-75\%}$
- Decreased FEV_T
- Decreased FEV_1/FVC ratio
- Decreased MVV
- Decreased PEFR
- Decreased $\dot{V}_{max\ 50}$

LUNG VOLUME AND CAPACITY FINDINGS (see page 47)
- Increased V_T
- Increased RV
- Increased RV/TLC ratio   *↑ volumes*
- Increased FRC
- Increased CV
- Decreased VC
- Decreased IRV
- Decreased ERV

INCREASED HEART RATE, CARDIAC OUTPUT, AND BLOOD PRESSURE (see page 57)

INCREASED ANTEROPOSTERIOR CHEST DIAMETER (BARREL CHEST) (see page 67)

PURSED-LIP BREATHING (see page 67)

USE OF ACCESSORY MUSCLES DURING INSPIRATION (see page 61)

USE OF ACCESSORY MUSCLES DURING EXPIRATION (see page 64)

ARTERIAL BLOOD GASES

EARLY STAGES OF AN ASTHMATIC EPISODE
ACUTE ALVEOLAR HYPERVENTILATION WITH HYPOXEMIA (see page 48)

- Pa_{O_2}: decreased
- Pa_{CO_2}: decreased
- HCO_3^-: decreased
- pH: increased

ADVANCED STAGES OF AN ASTHMATIC EPISODE (STATUS ASTHMATICUS)
ACUTE VENTILATORY FAILURE WITH HYPOXEMIA (see page 52)

- Pa_{O_2}: decreased
- Pa_{CO_2}: increased
- HCO_3^-: increased
- pH: decreased

CYANOSIS (see page 16)

COUGH AND SPUTUM PRODUCTION (see page 58)

CHEST ASSESSMENT FINDINGS (see page 3)

- Decreased tactile and vocal fremitus
- Hyperresonant percussion note
- Diminished breath sounds
- Crackles/rhonchi/wheezing

PULSUS PARADOXUS

When an asthmatic episode produces severe alveolar air trapping and hyperinflation, pulsus paradoxus is a classic clinical manifestation. Pulsus paradoxus is defined as a systolic blood pressure that is more than 10 mm Hg lower on inspiration than on expiration. This exaggerated waxing and waning of arterial blood pressure can be detected by using a sphygmomanometer or, in severe cases, by palpating the pulse. Pulsus paradoxus during an asthmatic attack is believed to be due to the major intrapleural pressure differences during inspiration and expiration.

DECREASED BLOOD PRESSURE DURING INSPIRATION

During inspiration, the patient frequently recruits accessory muscles of inspiration. The accessory muscles help to produce a greater negative intrapleural pressure, which in turn enhances intrapulmonary gas flow. The increased negative intrapleural pressure, however, also causes blood vessels in the lungs to dilate and to pool blood. Consequently, the volume of blood returning to the left ventricle decreases. This causes a reduction in cardiac output and arterial blood pressure during inspiration.

INCREASED BLOOD PRESSURE DURING EXPIRATION

During expiration, the patient often activates the accessory muscles of expiration in an effort to overcome the increased R_{aw}. The increased power produced by these accessory muscles of expiration generates a greater positive intrapleural pressure. Although increased positive intrapleural pressure helps to offset R_{aw}, it also works to narrow or squeeze the blood vessels of the lung. This increased pressure on the pulmonary blood vessels enhances left ventricular filling and results in an increased cardiac output and arterial blood pressure during expiration.

CHEST X-RAY FINDINGS

• Translucencies
• Depressed or flattened diaphragm

As the alveoli become enlarged during an asthmatic attack, the residual volume and functional residual capacity increase. This condition decreases the density of the lungs. Consequently, the x-ray films are translucent or darker than normal in appearance. Because of the increased residual volume and functional residual capacity, the diaphragm is depressed and flattened (Fig 5–4).

GENERAL MANAGEMENT OF ASTHMA

Environmental Control

The patient should make every effort to eliminate common household factors that may trigger an asthmatic episode. For example, rugs, drapes, furniture, and bed linen should be aired frequently. Foam rubber pillows should replace pillows made of feathers, and damp areas such as the basement should be well ventilated and kept dry. Other household members or visitors should not be allowed to smoke

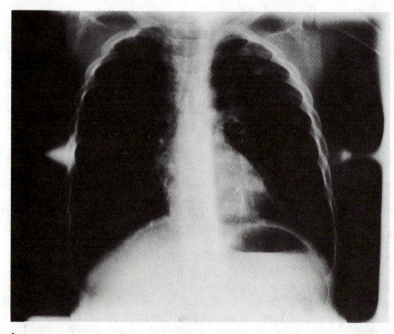

FIG 5–4.
Chest x-ray film of a 2-year-old patient during an asthmatic attack.

in the house. The heating system should be cleaned at least once a year, and temperature and humidity should be maintained at a comfortable level.

Medications

Sympathomimetics.—Sympathomimetic drugs are, perhaps, the most popular agents used in the treatment of asthma (see Appendix II).

Parasympatholytic Agents.—Parasympatholytic agents are also used to offset bronchial smooth muscle constriction (see Appendix III).

Xanthine Bronchodilators.—Xanthine bronchodilators are used to enhance bronchial smooth muscle relaxation (see Appendix IV).

Corticosteroids.—Although the exact mode of action of corticosteroids is not known, they have been shown to be very effective in treating asthma when other measures have failed (see Appendix V).

Mobilization of Bronchial Secretions

Because of the excessive mucus production and accumulation associated with asthma, a number of respiratory therapy modalities may be used to enhance the mobilization of bronchial secretions (see Appendix XI).

Supplemental Oxygen

Because of the hypoxemia associated with asthma, supplemental oxygen may be required. The hypoxemia that develops in asthma is most commonly caused by the hypoventilation and shuntlike effect associated with the disorder. Hypoxemia caused by a shuntlike effect can generally be corrected by oxygen therapy.

Monitoring

Arterial blood gases and some form of pulmonary function measurement such as PEFR or $FEF_{25\%-75\%}$ are used to assess the severity of the asthmatic episode. These measurements are made periodically to evaluate the patient's response to treatment. Vital signs must also be monitored closely, and a chest x-ray film should be obtained as soon as possible to help evaluate the degree of air trapping.

Mechanical Ventilation

Status asthmaticus is defined as a severe asthmatic episode that does not respond to bronchodilators. When these patients become fatigued, their respiratory rate decreases, and their arterial blood gases deteriorate. Clinically, the patient demonstrates a progressive decrease in Pa_{O_2} and pH and a steady increase in Pa_{CO_2}. If this trend is not reversed, mechanical ventilation becomes necessary.

situations, however, reading the questions and writing the answers down by themselves would be more efficient. If the a questionnaire is being completed by a respondent while the data collector is present, it is called an administered questionnaire. If the questionnaire is completed anonymously in a large group session, the interviewer effect could be significantly reduced. The questionnaire, however, need not be administered by the data collector. The respondents can take the questionnaire home and complete it at their convenience. Or the questionnaire can be mailed to the prospective respondents with a request for the respondents to send it back (usually a self-addressed envelop with postage paid is enclosed when sending out the questionnaire). The advantage of mailed questionnaires is that the interviewer effect is reduced to a minimum if no identification is attached. The disadvantage is that the response rate could also be significantly lowered.

Measurement is a key concern in a questionnaire. Nevertheless, questionnaire design needs to take into consideration more factors than the design of individual questions. The length of the entire questionnaire, the number of topics and types of questions included, the order of arranging the questions to be asked, and the patterns of the answers to be coded will all count. Generally speaking, a so-called close-ended question with all possible answers clarified and precoded appears more structured than an open-ended question. It is to your advantage in processing the data if you can make all your questions close-ended, unless it is essential to keep some of them open (without prescribing any answers or multiple choices).

SELF-ASSESSMENT QUESTIONS

Multiple Choice

1. During an asthmatic episode, the smooth muscle of the bronchi may hypertrophy as much as
   - a. 2 times normal size.
   - b. 3 times normal size.
   - c. 4 times normal size.
   - d. 5 times normal size.
   - e. 6 times normal size.

2. Asthma causes a/an
   - I. Increase in goblet cells.
   - II. Decrease in cilia.
   - III. Increase in bronchial gland size.
   - IV. Decrease in eosinophils.
     - a. I and III only.
     - b. II and IV only.
     - c. I, II, and III only.
     - d. II, III, and IV only.
     - e. I, II, III, and IV.

3. During an extrinsic-type asthma attack, the lymphoid tissue cells form which antibody?
   - a. IgA.
   - b. IgM.
   - c. IgG.
   - d. IgE.

4. When chemical mediators of the mast cells are released,
   - I. cAMP increases.
   - II. Bronchial constriction occurs.
   - III. Blood vessels constrict.
   - IV. Tissue edema occurs.
     - a. I only.
     - b. II only.
     - c. II and IV only.
     - d. I and III only.
     - e. I, III, and IV only.

5. When arranged for pressure (P), Poiseuille's law states that P is
   - I. Indirectly related to r^4
   - II. Directly related to $\dot{V}$
   - III. Indirectly related to l.
   - IV. Directly related to n.
     - a. I and III only.
     - b. II and IV only.
     - c. III and IV only.
     - d. I, II, and IV only.
     - e. II, III, and IV only.

6. When pulsus paradoxus appears during an asthma attack,
   - I. Left ventricle filling is increased during inspiration.
   - II. Cardiac output decreases during expiration.
   - III. Left ventricle filling increases during expiration.

IV. Cardiac output increases during inspiration.
   a. I only.
   b. II only.
   c. III only.
   d. I and II only.
   e. III and IV only.

7. During an asthmatic episode, the following abnormal lung volume and capacity findings are found:
   I. Increased FRC.
   II. Decreased ERV.
   III. Increased FEV_1.
   IV. Decreased CV.
      a. I only.
      b. II only.
      c. I and II only.
      d. III and IV only.
      e. II, III, and IV only.

8. During mast cell degranulation, which of the following chemical mediators are released?
   I. Bradykinin.
   II. ECF-A.
   III. Histamine.
   IV. SRS-A.
      a. I only.
      b. II only.
      c. III only.
      d. II and IV only.
      e. I, II, III, and IV.

9. Patients commonly present with these arterial blood gas values during an acute asthmatic episode:
   I. Increased pH.
   II. Increased Pa_{CO_2}.
   III. Decreased HCO_3^-.
   IV. Decreased Pa_{O_2}.
      a. IV only.
      b. I and III only.
      c. II and IV only.
      d. I, II, and III only.
      e. I, III, and IV only.

True or False

1. Pathologic alterations of the lungs are absent between asthmatic episodes.   True _____   False _____
2. A patient with extrinsic asthma generally demonstrates symptoms after the age of 30 years.   True _____   False _____
3. There is generally an absence of an antigen-antibody reaction in intrinsic asthma.   True _____   False _____
4. Extrinsic asthma is also known as an allergic disorder.   True _____   False _____
5. A partial β_2-blockade may be responsible for the occurrence of asthma in some individuals.   True _____   False _____
6. During an asthmatic attack, wheezing occurs more frequently during expiration.   True _____   False _____

Matching

Directions: On the line next to the trade name in column A, match the generic name from column B. Items in column B may be used once, more than once, or not at all.

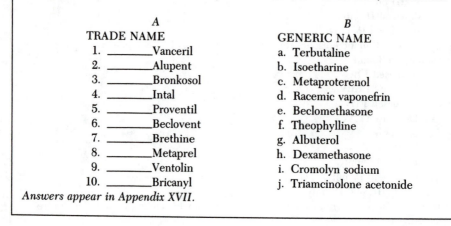

A	B
TRADE NAME	GENERIC NAME
1. _____Vanceril	a. Terbutaline
2. _____Alupent	b. Isoetharine
3. _____Bronkosol	c. Metaproterenol
4. _____Intal	d. Racemic vaponefrin
5. _____Proventil	e. Beclomethasone
6. _____Beclovent	f. Theophylline
7. _____Brethine	g. Albuterol
8. _____Metaprel	h. Dexamethasone
9. _____Ventolin	i. Cromolyn sodium
10. _____Bricanyl	j. Triamcinolone acetonide

Answers appear in Appendix XVII.

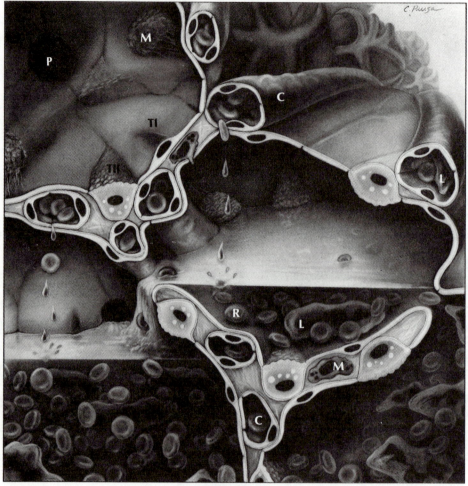

PNEUMONIA

FIG 6–1.
Alveolar consolidation in pneumonia. *P* = pore of Kohn; *M* = macrophage; *TI* = type I cell; *TII* = type II cell; *C* = capillary; *L* = leukocyte; *R* = red blood cell.

PNEUMONIA

ANATOMIC ALTERATIONS OF THE LUNGS

Pneumonia, or pneumonitis with consolidation, is an inflammatory process that primarily affects the gas exchange area of the lung. In response to the inflammation, fluid (serum) and some red blood cells (RBCs) from adjacent pulmonary capillaries pour into the alveoli. This fluid transfer is called effusion. Polymorphonuclear leukocytes also move into the infected area to engulf and kill invading bacteria on the alveolar walls. This process has been termed "surface phagocytosis." Increased numbers of macrophages also appear in the infected area to remove cellular and bacterial debris. If the infection is overwhelming, the alveoli become completely filled with fluid, RBCs, polymorphonuclear leukocytes, and macrophages. When this occurs, the alveoli are said to be consolidated (Fig 6–1).

To summarize, the major pathologic or structural changes associated with pneumonia are as follows:

- Inflammation of the alveoli
- Alveolar consolidation

ETIOLOGY

The major causes of pneumonia are listed in Table 6–1 and are discussed in detail in this section.

Bacterial Causes

Gram-Positive Organisms

Streptococcal Pneumonia.—*Streptococcus pneumoniae* (formerly called *Diplococcus pneumoniae*) accounts for about 90% of all bacterial pneumonias. The organism is a gram-positive, nonmotile coccus that is found singly, in pairs, and in short chains (Fig 6–2).

There are more than 80 types of *Streptococcus pneumoniae*, but only 14 cause serious illness. Type 3 is the most commonly found pathogen in pneumonia.

Streptococci are generally transmitted by aerosol from a cough or a sneeze of an infected individual. Only very rarely is the organism transmitted by direct contact with contaminated objects.

TABLE 6–1.
Major Causes of Pneumonia

Bacterial causes	Other causes
Gram-positive organisms	*Mycoplasma pneumoniae*
Streptococcus	Rickettsial infections
Staphylococcus	Ornithosis
Gram-negative organisms	Varicella
Klebsiella	Rubella
Pseudomonas aeruginosa	Aspiration of gastric content
Haemophilus influenzae	Aspiration of lipids
Legionella	Pneumocystosis
Viral causes	
Influenza virus	
Respiratory syncytial virus	
Parainfluenza virus	
Adenovirus	

Staphylococcal Pneumonia.—There are two major groups of staphylococci: (1) *Staphylococcus aureus*, which is responsible for most "staph" infections in humans, and (2) *Staphylococcus albus* and/or *epidermidis*, which is part of the normal flora.

The staphylococci are gram-positive cocci that are found singly, in pairs, and in irregular clusters (Fig 6–3).

Staphylococcal pneumonia often follows a predisposing virus infection. *Staphylococcus aureus* is commonly transmitted by aerosol from a cough or sneeze of an infected individual and indirectly via contact with floors, bedding, contaminated clothes, and the like.

Gram-Negative Organisms

The major gram-negative organisms responsible for pneumonia are rod-shaped microorganisms called bacilli (Fig 6–4).

Klebsiella Pneumoniae *(Friedländer's bacillus).*—*Klebsiella pneumoniae* has long been associated with lobar pneumonia, particularly in men over 40 years old and in chronic alcoholics of both sexes. *Klebsiella* is a gram-negative bacillus that is found singly, in pairs, or in chains of varying lengths. It is a normal inhabitant of the human gastrointestinal tract.

The organism can be transmitted directly by aerosol or indirectly by contact

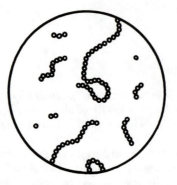

FIG 6–2.
The streptococcus organism is a gram-positive, nonmotile coccus that is found singly, in pairs, and in short chains.

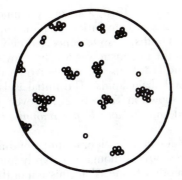

FIG 6–3.
The staphylococcus organism is a gram-positive, nonmotile coccus that is found singly, in pairs, and in irregular clusters.

with freshly contaminated articles. The mortality of patients with *Klebsiella* pneumonia has been quite high since septicemia is a frequent complication.

Pseudomonas Aeruginosa *Pneumonia* (Bacillus pyocyaneus).—*Pseudomonas aeruginosa* is a highly motile, gram-negative bacillus. It is found in the human gastrointestinal tract and is a contaminant in many aqueous solutions. It is frequently cultured from the respiratory tract of chronically ill, tracheotomized patients. This makes *Pseudomonas aeruginosa* a particular problem to the respiratory therapy practitioner. Since the *Pseudomonas* organism thrives in dampness, it is frequently cultured from contaminated respiratory therapy equipment.

The sputum from patients with *Pseudomonas* infection is frequently green and sweet smelling. The organism is commonly transmitted by aerosol or by direct contact with freshly contaminated articles.

Haemophilus Influenzae *Pneumonia*.—*Haemophilus influenzae* is frequently a cause of a secondary type of pneumonia following a primary viral infection. *Haemophilus influenzae* is one of the smallest gram-negative bacilli, measuring about 1.5 μm in length and 0.3 μm in width. There are six types of *Haemophilus influenzae*, designated A to F, but only type B is commonly pathogenic. The disease is often seen in children between the ages of 1 month and 6 years. The organism is transmitted via aerosol or contact with contaminated objects, but it is sensitive to cold and does not survive long after expectoration.

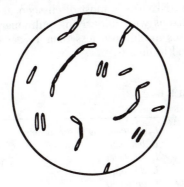

FIG 6–4.
The bacilli are rod-shaped microorganisms and the major gram-negative organisms responsible for pneumonia.

Legionella Pneumonia.—In July, 1976, a severe pneumonia-like disease outbreak occurred at an American Legion convention in Philadelphia. The causative agent eluded isolation for many months, despite concerted efforts of the nation's top epidemiologic experts. When the organism was finally recovered from a patient, it was found to be an unusual and fastidious gram-negative bacillus with atypical concentrations of certain branched-chain lipids. The initial isolate was designated as *Legionella pneumophila*. As shown in Table 6–2, however, there are presently seven different species identified, and *Legionella pneumophila* is now known to consist of six different serogroups.

The organism can be detected in pleural fluid, sputum, or lung tissue by direct fluorescent antibody microscopy. Although it is rarely found outside the lungs, the organism may be found in other tissue. Transmission of the disease is still not completely clear. It is believed, however, that a common source is the probable cause since it has been found in surface water, mud, and water from air conditioners. There is no direct evidence that the disease spreads from person to person. The disease is most commonly seen in middle-aged males who smoke. The mortality rate is between 15% and 25%.

Viral Causes

Viruses are minute organisms not visible by ordinary light microscopy. They are parasitic and depend on nutrients inside cells for their metabolic and reproductive needs. About 90% of acute upper respiratory tract infections and 50% of lower respiratory tract infections are due to viruses. The most common viruses causing respiratory infections are described below.

Influenza Virus.—The major subtypes of the influenza virus are A_0, A_1, A_2, B, and C. The A and B varieties rank as the primary causes of epidemic respiratory tract infections. Influenza A has also been found in horses, swine, and birds. Influenza viruses have an incubation period of 1 to 3 days. Transmission of the disease is by aerosol.

Influenza viruses cause mainly upper respiratory tract infections. Young adults in robust health appear to be particularly susceptible.

Respiratory Syncytial Virus.—The respiratory syncytial virus is a member of the paramyxovirus group. Parainfluenza, mumps, and rubeola viruses also belong to this group.

The respiratory syncytial virus is most often seen in children under 6 months of age and in elderly persons with underlying pulmonary disease. Approximately 25% of respiratory illnesses in children less than 1 year old are due to this virus. The infection is rarely fatal in infants.

TABLE 6–2.
Legionella Species

L. pneumophila (6 serogroups)
L. bozemanii
L. micdadei
L. dumoffii
L. gormanii
L. longbeachae
L. jordanis

The respiratory syncytial virus often goes unrecognized but may play an important role as a forerunner to bacterial infections. The virus is generally transmitted by aerosol and by direct contact with infected individuals.

Parainfluenza Virus.—The parainfluenza viruses are also members of the paramyxovirus group and therefore are related to mumps, rubella, and the respiratory syncytial viruses.

There are five types of parainfluenza viruses: types 1, 2, 3, 4A, and 4B. Types 1, 2, and 3 are the major causes of infections in humans. Type 1 is considered a "croup" type of virus. Types 2 and 3 are associated with severe infections. Although type 3 is seen in persons of all ages, it is most commonly seen in infants less than 2 months old. Types 1 and 2 are most often seen in children between the ages of 6 months and 5 years. Types 1 and 2 infections typically occur in the fall, while type 3 infection is most often seen in the late spring and summer. Parainfluenza viruses are transmitted by aerosol, and the virus spreads rapidly among members of the same family.

Adenoviruses.—There are at least 33 serologic adenovirus subgroups. Serotypes 1, 2, 3, 4, 5, and 7 are responsible for the most serious infections. About 60% of all adenovirus infections are caused by serotypes 1 and 2. Serotype 7 has been related to fatal cases of pneumonia in children. Adenoviruses are transmitted by aerosol and nasopharyngeal secretions from infected individuals.

Other Causes

Mycoplasma Pneumoniae.—The mycoplasmas are small, cell wall–deficient organisms. They are smaller than bacteria but larger than viruses. Their cell walls lack peptidoglycan. The pneumonia caused by the mycoplasmal organism is described as primary atypical pneumonia, atypical because the organism escapes isolation by standard bacteriologic tests.

Mycoplasma pneumoniae infection is not highly communicable. It may take weeks for the organism to spread, even among members of the same family. It is most frequently seen in adolescents and young adults.

Rickettsiae.—Rickettsiae are small, pleomorphic coccobacilli. Most rickettsiae are intracellular parasites possessing both RNA and DNA. There are several pathogenic members of the Rickettsia family: *Rickettsia rickettsii* (Rocky Mountain spotted fever), *Rickettsia akari* (rickettsialpox), *Rickettsia prowazekii* (typhus), and *Rickettsia burnetii*, also called *Coxiella burnetii* (Queensland [Q] fever).

All species of the genus *Rickettsia* are unstable outside of cells except for *Rickettsia burnetii* (Q fever), which is extremely resistant to heat and light. Q fever can cause a pneumonia as well as a prolonged febrile illness, an influenza-like illness, and endocarditis. The organism is commonly transmitted by arthropods (lice, fleas, ticks, mites). It may also be transmitted by cattle, sheep, and goats and possibly in raw milk.

Ornithosis (Psittacosis).—Ornithosis is an acute pulmonary infection caused by an organism of the *Chlamydia* or *Bedsonia* group. These are larger and more complex organisms than viruses and contain both DNA and RNA.

The organism is transmitted by many kinds of birds (parrots, parakeets, lorikeets, cockatoos, chickens, pigeons, ducks, pheasants, and turkeys) and from birds to humans via aerosol or by direct contact.

CHAPTER NINE

Triangulation and Modes of Research

So far, we have discussed different methods of data collection, and clarified some major issues that would characterize a research project. You may, however, be a little overwhelmed by the plethora of behavioral and social science research methods. In real terms, students often feel at a loss as research methods texts fail to supply a comprehensive scheme for them to put various methods and techniques in place. Indeed, some authors of research texts are quite at liberty to list together all kinds of designs, strategies, approaches, procedures, techniques, programs, and modes. What would really help the students to master the all too complex and complicated research business, however, is to let them have a systems perspective differentiating between different levels, dimensions, and subsystems of this bewildering universe. Nobody should confine himself nor confuse the system by ignoring the deep-seated structure of human inquiry. Rather, the individual researcher can optimize his research design by organizing a project around his substantive interests and/or methodological emphases. Here the appropriate way of "triangulation" takes the central stage. It means the pursuit of research in a multi-method, multi-faceted, systematic, and skillful manner. The following discussion will give you some clues about various research modes with the intention to point you to a higher level of mastery.

Addressing your purpose by every good means

Since science gained its position as an important institution in our society, it has formed its own tradition. This tradition marked the epoch-making progress in

Varicella (Chickenpox).—The varicella virus usually causes a benign disease in children between the ages of 2 and 8 years, and complications of varicella are not common. In some cases, however, varicella has been noted to spread to the lungs and cause a serious secondary pneumonitis.

Rubella (Measles).—Measles virus spreads from person to person by the respiratory route. Respiratory complications are often encountered in this disease because of widespread involvement of the mucosa of the respiratory tract.

Aspiration Pneumonitis.—Aspiration of gastric juice with a pH of 2.5 or less causes a serious and often fatal pneumonia. Aspiration pneumonitis is commonly missed since acute inflammatory reactions may not begin until several hours after aspiration of the gastric juice. The inflammatory reactions generally increase in severity for 12 to 26 hours. In the absence of a secondary bacterial infection, the inflammation usually becomes clinically insignificant in about 72 hours, although adult respiratory distress syndrome may develop in severe cases. Mendelson in 1946 first described the clinical manifestations of tachycardia, dyspnea, and cyanosis associated with the aspiration of acid stomach contents. The clinical picture he described is now known as the Mendelson's syndrome and is usually confined to aspiration pneumonitis in the parturient female.

Lipoid Pneumonitis.—The aspiration of mineral oil, used medically as a lubricant, has also been known to cause pneumonitis. The severity of the pneumonia is dependent on the type of oil aspirated. Oils from animal fats cause the most serious reaction, while oils of vegetable origin are relatively inert. When mineral oil is inhaled in an aerosolized form, an intense pulmonary tissue reaction occurs.

Pneumocystosis.—In severely immunosuppressed patients, the protozoan *Pneumocystis carinii* causes a form of pneumonia called pneumocystosis. Although it was once considered a clinical rarity, this infection is now being diagnosed with greater frequency. For example, pneumocystosis is the most common life-threatening infection in patients with the acquired immunodeficiency syndrome (AIDS) and appears in nearly 60% of cases.

OVERVIEW OF THE CARDIOPULMONARY CLINICAL MANIFESTATIONS ASSOCIATED WITH PNEUMONIA

INCREASED RESPIRATORY RATE
Several pathophysiologic mechanisms operating simultaneously may lead to an increased ventilatory rate. These are (see page 23):

• Stimulation of peripheral chemoreceptors
• Decreased lung compliance/increased work of breathing relationship
• Stimulation of the J receptors
• Pain/anxiety

PULMONARY FUNCTION STUDIES

LUNG VOLUME AND CAPACITY FINDINGS (see page 37)
• Decreased VC
• Decreased RV
• Decreased FRC

- Decreased TLC
- Decreased V$_T$

INCREASED HEART RATE, CARDIAC OUTPUT, AND BLOOD PRESSURE (see page 57)

ARTERIAL BLOOD GASES

EARLY STAGES OF PNEUMONIA
ACUTE ALVEOLAR HYPERVENTILATION WITH HYPOXEMIA (see page 48)

- Pa$_{O_2}$: decreased
- Pa$_{CO_2}$: decreased
- HCO$_3^-$: decreased
- pH: increased

ADVANCED STAGES OF PNEUMONIA
ACUTE VENTILATORY FAILURE WITH HYPOXEMIA (see page 52)

- Pa$_{O_2}$: decreased
- Pa$_{CO_2}$: increased
- HCO$_3^-$: increased
- pH: decreased

CYANOSIS (see page 16)

PLEURAL EFFUSION (see Chapter 12)

CHEST ASSESSMENT FINDINGS (see page 3)

- Increased tactile and vocal fremitus
- Dull percussion note
- Bronchial breath sounds
- Crackles/rhonchi
- Pleural friction rub
- Whispered pectoriloquy

COUGH, SPUTUM PRODUCTION, AND HEMOPTYSIS (see page 58)

Initially, a patient with pneumonia usually has a nonproductive barking or hacking cough. As the disease progresses, the cough usually becomes productive of purulent, blood-streaked, or rusty sputum. This is caused by fluid moving from the pulmonary capillaries into the alveoli in response to the inflammatory process. As fluid crosses into the alveoli, some RBCs will also move into the alveoli and produce the blood-streaked or rusty appearance of the fluid (see Fig 6–1).

As the disease progresses, some of the fluid that moves into the alveoli will also work its way into the bronchioles and bronchi. As the fluid accumulates in the bronchial tree, the subepithelial mechanoreceptors located in the trachea, bronchi, and bronchioles are stimulated and initiate a cough reflex.

Since bronchioles and bronchi are deep in the lung parenchyma, the patient with pneumonia initially has a dry, hacking cough, and fluid cannot be easily expectorated until the process involves the larger bronchi.

CHEST PAIN/DECREASED CHEST EXPANSION (see page 70)

CHEST X-RAY FINDINGS

- Increased density
- Consolidation and atelectasis
- Air bronchograms
- Pleural effusions

Because of the numerous causes of pneumonia, the radiographic signs vary considerably. In general, pneumonia appears as an area of increased density that may involve a small lung segment, a lobe, a lung, or both lungs (Fig 6–5). As the alveoli become consolidated, the density increases. Air bronchograms, atelectasis, and pleural effusion are often seen. Clinically, the radiographic signs of pneumonia are very similar to those produced in cardiogenic pulmonary edema.

GENERAL MANAGEMENT OF PNEUMONIA

Hyperinflation Techniques

Hyperinflation measures are commonly ordered to offset the alveolar consolidation associated with pneumonia (see Appendix XII).

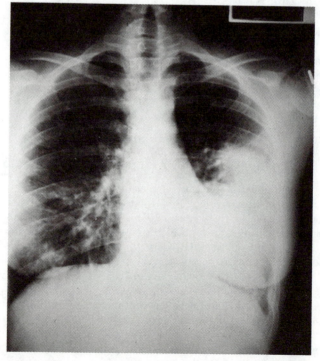

FIG 6–5.
Chest x-ray film of a 20-year-old woman with a severe left-lung pneumonia.

Medications

Antibiotic Agents.—Antibiotics are commonly used to combat the infectious agents causing the pneumonia (see Appendix VIII).

Analgesic Agents.—Analgesics may be ordered to relieve pleuritic pain. As the pain decreases, the depth of inspiration and cough effort should improve.

Aerosolized Pentamidine.—Pentamidine has antiprotozoal activity and has been found to be effective against *Pneumocystis carinii.*

Supplemental Oxygen

Because of the hypoxemia associated with pneumonia, supplemental oxygen may be required. It should be noted, however, that the hypoxemia that develops in pneumonia is most commonly caused by the alveolar consolidation and capillary shunting associated with the disorder. Hypoxemia caused by capillary shunting is often refractory to oxygen therapy.

Thoracentesis

A thoracentesis is commonly performed when pleural effusion develops from pneumonia. The fluid is generally analyzed for the following:

- Color
- Odor
- RBC count
- WBC count with differential
- Protein
- Sugar
- Lactic dehydrogenase (LDH)
- Amylase
- pH
- Wright, Gram, and acid-fast (AFB) stains
- Aerobic, anaerobic, tuberculosis, and fungal cultures
- Cytology

SELF-ASSESSMENT QUESTIONS

Multiple Choice

1. Which of the following is known as Friedländer's bacillus?
   a. *Haemophilus influenzae.*
   b. *Pseudomonas aeruginosa.*
   c. *Legionella.*
   d. *Klebsiella.*
   e. *Streptococcus.*
2. Of the six types of *Haemophilus influenzae,* which type is most frequently pathogenic?
   a. Type A.
   b. Type B.

   c. Type C.
   d. Type D.
   e. Type E.
   f. Type F.
3. Which of the following virus(es) is/are a member of the paramyxovirus group?
   I. Influenza virus.
   II. Respiratory syncytial virus.
   III. Parainfluenza virus.
   IV. Adenovirus.
      a. II only.
      b. IV only.
      c. I and II only.
      d. II and III only.
      e. II, III, and IV only.
4. Which of the following is associated with Q fever?
      a. *Mycoplasma pneumoniae*.
      b. *Rickettsia*.
      c. Ornithosis.
      d. Varicella.
      e. Respiratory syncytial virus.
5. Mendelson is associated with
      a. Lipoid pneumonitis.
      b. Rubella.
      c. Varicella.
      d. Aspiration pneumonitis.
      e. *Rickettsia*.
6. Pneumonia causes which of the following?
   I. Shunt effect.
   II. Physiologic dead space.
   III. Venous admixture.
   IV. Anatomic dead space.
      a. I and II only.
      b. II and III only.
      c. III and IV only.
      d. II and IV only.
      e. I and III only.
7. A patient with acute pneumonia commonly has the following arterial blood gas values:
   I. Increased pH.
   II. Increased Pa_{CO_2}.
   III. Increased HCO_3^-.
   IV. Increased Pa_{O_2}.
      a. I only.
      b. II only.
      c. III and IV only.
      d. I, II, and III only.
      e. II, III, and IV only.
8. The bulk of CO_2 produced in the tissue cells is transported to the lungs as
      a. Carbonic acid (H_2CO_3).
      b. Bicarbonate (HCO_3^-).
      c. Dissolved CO_2 in plasma.
      d. Carbaminohemoglobin.
      e. Carbonic anhydrase.

9. In the absence of a secondary bacterial infection, lung inflammation caused by the aspiration of gastric fluids usually becomes insignificant in about
   a. 2 days.
   b. 3 days.
   c. 5 days.
   d. 7 days.
   e. 10 days.

True or False

1. Approximately 90% of all bacterial pneumonias are caused by the streptococcus organism.   True _____   False _____
2. The streptococcus organism is a gram-negative organism.   True _____   False _____
3. *Staphylococcus aureus* is responsible for most staph infections in humans.   True _____   False _____
4. About 90% of acute upper respiratory tract infections are due to viruses.   True _____   False _____
5. Type 1 parainfluenza virus is considered a "croup" virus.   True _____   False _____
6. The increased pH level noted in acute pneumonia occurs as a result of a decreased Pa_{CO_2}.   True _____   False _____
7. The chest pain sometimes noted in pneumonia is often due to fluid irritation of the visceral pleura.   True _____   False _____
8. Gentamicin is an effective drug in treating a pneumonia caused by *Pseudomonas aeruginosa*.   True _____   False _____
9. Ampicillin is an effective drug in treating a pneumonia caused by *Haemophilus influenzae*.   True _____   False _____
10. Penicillin G is an effective drug in treating a pneumonia caused by a parainfluenza virus.   True _____   False _____

Answers appear in Appendix XVII.

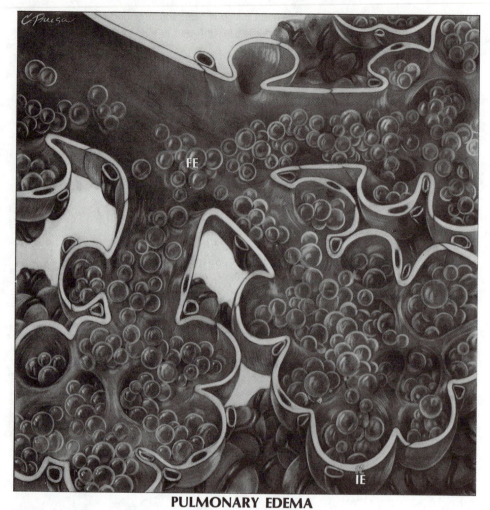

PULMONARY EDEMA

FIG 7–1.
Pulmonary edema. *FE* = frothy edema; *IE* = interstitial edema.

• 7

PULMONARY EDEMA

ANATOMIC ALTERATIONS OF THE LUNGS

Pulmonary edema is an excessive movement of fluid from the pulmonary vascular system to the extravascular system and air spaces of the lungs. Fluid first seeps into the perivascular and peribronchial interstitial spaces and, depending on the degree of severity, progressively moves into the alveoli, bronchioles, and bronchi.

As a consequence of this fluid movement, the alveolar wall interstitium widens, and an increase in the surface tension causes the swollen alveoli to shrink in size. Moreover, much of the fluid that accumulates in the tracheobronchial tree is churned into a frothy sputum as a result of air moving in and out of the lungs. The abundance of fluid in the interstitial spaces causes the lymphatic vessels to widen and the lymph flow to increase (Fig 7–1).

The major pathologic or structural changes associated with pulmonary edema are summarized as follows:

- Interstitial edema, including fluid engorgement of the perivascular and peribronchial spaces and the alveolar wall interstitium
- Increased surface tension
- Alveolar shrinkage
- Frothy secretions throughout the tracheobronchial tree

ETIOLOGY

The etiology of pulmonary edema can be divided into two major categories, cardiogenic and noncardiogenic.

Cardiogenic Pulmonary Edema

Ordinarily, hydrostatic pressure of about 10 to 15 mm Hg tends to move fluid out of the pulmonary capillaries into the interstitial space. This force is normally offset by colloid osmotic forces of about 25 to 30 mm Hg that tend to keep fluid in the pulmonary capillaries. The colloid osmotic pressure is referred to as *oncotic pressure* and is produced by the albumin and globulin particles in the blood. The stability of fluid within the pulmonary capillaries is therefore determined by the balance between hydrostatic and oncotic pressure. This hydrostatic and oncotic relationship also maintains fluid stability in the interstitial compartments.

Movement of fluid in and out of the capillaries is expressed by Starling's equation:

$$J = K (Pc - Pi) - (\pi c - \pi i)$$

where J is the net fluid movement out of the capillary, K is the capillary permeability factor, Pc and Pi are the hydrostatic pressures in the capillary and interstitial space, and πc and πi are the oncotic pressures in the capillary and interstitial space.

Though conceptually valuable, this equation has limited practical use. Of the four pressures, only the oncotic and hydrostatic pressures of the pulmonary capillaries can be identified with any certainty. The oncotic and hydrostatic pressures within the interstitial compartments cannot be readily determined.

When the hydrostatic pressure within the pulmonary vascular system rises to more than 25 to 30 mm Hg, the oncotic pressure loses its holding force over the fluid within the pulmonary capillaries. Consequently, fluid will start to spill into the interstitial and air spaces of the lungs.

Increased hydrostatic pressure is considered the most common cause of pulmonary edema. In alphabetical order, some causes of cardiogenic pulmonary edema are as follows:

• Arrhythmias
• Excessive fluid administration
• Left ventricular failure
• Mitral valve disease
• Myocardial infarction
• Pulmonary embolus
• Renal failure
• Rheumatic heart disease (myocarditis)
• Systemic hypertension

Noncardiogenic Pulmonary Edema

Increased Capillary Permeability.—Pulmonary edema may develop due to increased capillary permeability as a result of infectious, inflammatory, and other processes. The following are some causes of increased capillary permeability:

• Alveolar hypoxia
• Adult respiratory distress syndrome
• Inhalation of toxic agents such as chlorine, sulfur dioxide, nitrogen oxides, ammonia, and phosgene
• Pneumonia
• Therapeutic radiation of the lungs

Lymphatic Insufficiency.—Should the lungs' normal lymphatic drainage be decreased, intravascular and extravascular fluid begins to pool, and pulmonary edema ensues. Lymphatic drainage may be slowed because of obliteration or distortion of lymphatic vessels. The lymphatic vessels may be obstructed by tumor cells in lymphangitis carcinomatosa. Because the lymphatic vessels empty into systemic veins, increased systemic venous pressure may slow lymphatic drainage. Lymphatic insufficiency has also been observed following lung transplantation.

Decreased Intrapleural Pressure.—Reduced intrapleural pressure may cause pulmonary edema. During severe airway obstruction, for example, the negative pressure exerted by the patient during inspiration may create a suction effect on the pulmonary capillaries and cause fluid to move into the alveoli.

Furthermore, the increased negative intrapleural pressure promotes filling of the right heart and hinders left-heart blood flow. This condition may cause pooling of blood in the lungs and, subsequently, an elevated hydrostatic pressure and pulmonary edema.

Decreased Oncotic Pressure.—Although this condition is rare, if the oncotic pressure is reduced from its normal 25 to 30 mm Hg and falls below the patient's normal hydrostatic pressure of 10 to 15 mm Hg, fluid will begin to seep into the interstitial and air spaces of the lungs. Decreased oncotic pressure may be caused by the following:

- Overtransfusion and/or rapid transfusion of intravenous fluid
- Uremia
- Hypoproteinemia
- Acute nephritis
- Polyarteritis nodosa

Other Causes

Although the exact mechanisms are not known, pulmonary edema can also be caused by the following:

- Allergic reaction to drugs
- Aspiration
- Central nervous system (CNS) stimulation
- Cerebral hemorrhage
- Encephalitis
- Heroin overdosage
- Skull trauma

OVERVIEW OF THE CARDIOPULMONARY CLINICAL MANIFESTATIONS ASSOCIATED WITH PULMONARY EDEMA

INCREASED RESPIRATORY RATE

Several pathophysiologic mechanisms operating simultaneously may lead to an increased ventilatory rate. These are (see page 23):

- Stimulation of peripheral chemoreceptors
- Decreased lung compliance/increased work of breathing relationship
- Stimulation of the J receptors
- Anxiety

not relate to the students' immediate needs. Without a comprehensive and dialectic understanding of the research process, the students would find it difficult to get the points and grasp the essence of various parts. Even if they have attained such an understanding through long-term endeavor, the researchers will need something as comprehensive as a handbook and as succinct as an outline for periodic review in order to keep or regain that understanding after some years in practice.

Moreover, there are practical issues in research to which the textbooks are usually not in a position to provide even tentative answers. As a former student and a current instructor in research, I have keenly felt the need for a book that does not simply repeat the available literature, but provides a practical guide to the mastery of this extremely important subject. Such a guide should address the real issues a student would face and view them with the student's eyes. It should be able to serve as a core text to suit the needs of those instructors who desire to amplify their courses with other paperbacks and their own materials.

This book is intended to be such a guide and core reading by speaking from a student's experience. It organizes behavioral and social research methods in a manner most relevant to the student and explains them in a plain language. It is aimed at helping the reader to approach research with vision and confidence. The guide is especially written for those students who have a thesis and/or dissertation to write for their intended academic/professional degree(s). To write the thesis or dissertation they must undertake a research project of their own. The thesis or dissertation is supposed to demonstrate their mastery of the substantive field as well as the needed research skills. And more often than not, it is expected to contribute something new or "original" to the knowledge body as defined immediately by their thesis or dissertation committee, and in the long run by all the experts who happen to read it.

In real terms, the thesis or dissertation provides a unique research experience. As a process of intensive training it would transform the student into a genuine researcher and scientist. And the results of the thesis/dissertation research oftentimes set a milestone for the entire career of the student. As part of the human undertaking in scientific inquiry, the thesis/dissertation research could make a significant difference in our knowledge and understanding. Many of those who have successfully obtained their degree(s), however, have the regret of failing to publish their thesis and/or dissertation. This book will show you, also speaking from a student's real experience, how to write a publishable thesis or dissertation and eventually get it published.

(A note to the instructor: Lecture may begin with chapter five. Other topics can be added as needed.)

human history, yet could not help creating new shackles for science itself. The orthodox scientific method has been defined by reduction, quantification, and hypothesis testing, while other forms of human inquiry have not appealed to the delicate methodological taste. In recent years, however, behavioral and social scientists have witnessed many alternative approaches coming to the fore, with the revitalization of some "primitive" methods in human inquiry. Many of the alternative approaches and methods are used, transmitted, and taught under the rubric of "qualitative research" as opposed to the traditional quantitative methods. Instead of talking about operationalization and statistical hypothesis testing, qualitative methods emphasize interpretive, descriptive, narrative and other artistically grounded approaches to research. In many cases, qualitative research has helped frame the situation and ask the question, if not in generalizing the conclusion. Indeed, one can hardly imagine that behavioral and social sciences could make all the progresses by solely relying on the orthodox, positivist research paradigm. In discussing the modes of research, therefore, we need to take into consideration all forms of inquiry, alternatively structured or even unstructured, that contribute to the scientific understanding of human life. Theoretical reasoning is certainly an important form or link of research, but here we are more concerned with the collection and analysis of empirical data, which can be quantified (quantitative data) or not quantified (qualitative data).

To see how different sources and types of data as well as different research methods may serve the same purpose, let us look at two important modes of current social research, respectively. The first is called historical/comparative study, and the second, evaluation research. Both modes involve group comparison as a central piece of the research design, and embrace a longitudinal process or historical perspective in gathering and processing the data. The difference is in that the historical/comparative study usually has a broader scope that may go across different cultures and nations, and an extended time horizon that may cover years, decades, or even centuries. An evaluation research, in contrast, is usually limited within a part or some parts of a country and within a relatively short period of time. Another difference is that historical/comparative study tends to use unobtrusive measures or indirect data such as existing statistics for large-scale analysis, whereas evaluation research usually relies on direct data collection and is often tied with some sort of intervention. In addition, evaluation research tends to be more quantitative-oriented while historical/comparative study may include more qualitative data. Of course, this is not to say that the two research modes will use absolutely different methods, nor that the two different

PULMONARY FUNCTION STUDIES

LUNG VOLUME AND CAPACITY FINDINGS (see page 37)
- Decreased VC
- Decreased RV
- Decreased FRC
- Decreased TLC
- Decreased V_T

ARTERIAL BLOOD GASES

EARLY STAGES OF PULMONARY EDEMA
ACUTE ALVEOLAR HYPERVENTILATION WITH HYPOXEMIA (see page 48)
- Pa_{O_2}: decreased
- Pa_{CO_2}: decreased
- HCO_3^-: decreased
- pH: increased

ADVANCED STAGES OF PULMONARY EDEMA
ACUTE VENTILATORY FAILURE WITH HYPOXEMIA (see page 52)
- Pa_{O_2}: decreased
- Pa_{CO_2}: increased
- HCO_3^-: increased
- pH: decreased

CYANOSIS (see page 16)

COUGH AND SPUTUM PRODUCTION (FROTHY) (see page 58)

CHEST ASSESSMENT FINDINGS (see page 3)

- Increased tactile and vocal fremitus
- Crackles/rhonchi/wheezing

PLEURAL EFFUSION (see Chapter 12)

PAROXYSMAL NOCTURNAL DYSPNEA

Patients with pulmonary edema often awaken with severe dyspnea after several hours of sleep. This is particularly true of patients with cardiogenic pulmonary edema. While the patient is awake, more time is spent in the erect position, and as a result, excess fluids tend to accumulate in the dependent portions of the body. When the patient lies down, however, the excess fluid from the peripheral parts of the body move into the blood stream and cause an increase in venous return to the lungs. This action raises the pulmonary capillary pressure and promotes pulmonary edema. The pulmonary edema in turn promotes pulmonary shunting, venous admixture, and hypoxemia. When the hypoxemia becomes severe, the peripheral chemoreceptors are stimulated and initiate an increased ventilatory rate (see Fig 1–52). The decreased lung compliance, J receptor stimulation, and anxiety may also contribute to the paroxysmal nocturnal dyspnea commonly noted in this disorder. A patient is said to have orthopnea when dyspnea increases while the patient is in a recumbent position.

INCREASED PULMONARY WEDGE PRESSURE

A flow-directed (Swan-Ganz) catheter is often placed into the pulmonary artery to differentiate between cardiogenic and noncardiogenic pulmonary edema. In patients with left-sided heart failure, the pulmonary wedge pressure is high (>20 to 25 mm Hg). In patients with noncardiogenic pulmonary edema, the pulmonary wedge pressure is usually within normal limits (about 10 to 15 mm Hg).

CHEST X-RAY FINDINGS

- Fluffy opacity
- Ventricular hypertrophy
- Kerley B lines
- Pleural effusion

CARDIOGENIC

Since x-ray densities reflect primarily alveolar filling and not interstitial edema, by the time abnormal findings are encountered the pathologic changes associated with pulmonary edema are advanced. Chest x-ray films typically reveal dense, fluffy opacities that spread outward from the hilar areas to the peripheral borders of the lungs (Fig 7–2,A). The peripheral portion of the lungs often remains clear, and this produces what is described as a "butterfly" or "batwing" distribution. Left ventricular hypertrophy and enlarged pulmonary vessels are commonly seen. Pleural effusions may be seen. Finally, Kerley B lines may appear on the radiograph as a result of the interstitial edema. The lines are short, straight markings that originate near the pleural surface of the lower regions of the lungs. They are thought to be caused by edematous interlobular septa (Fig 7–2,B).

NONCARDIOGENIC

In noncardiogenic pulmonary edema, the chest x-ray film commonly shows areas of fluffy densities that are usually more dense near the hilum. The density may be unilateral or bilateral. Pleural effusion is usually not present, and the cardiac silhouette is not enlarged.

GENERAL MANAGEMENT OF PULMONARY EDEMA

Hyperinflation Techniques

Hyperinflation measures are commonly ordered to offset the fluid accumulation and alveolar shrinkage associated with pulmonary edema (see Appendix XII).

Supplemental Oxygen

Because of the hypoxemia associated with pulmonary edema, supplemental oxygen may be required. It should be noted, however, that the hypoxemia that develops in pulmonary edema is most commonly caused by the alveolar fluid and cap-

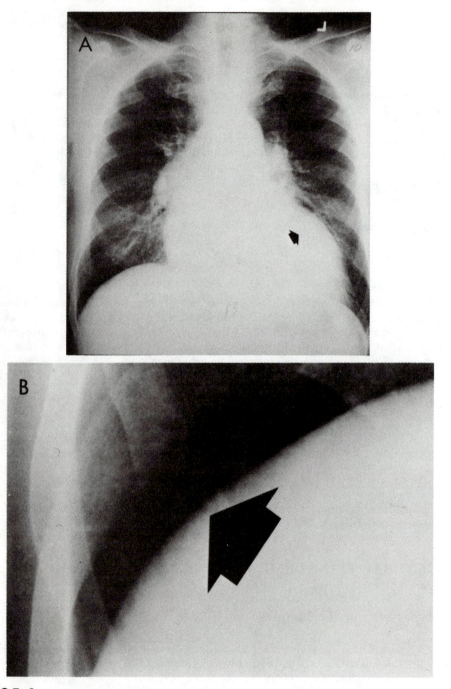

FIG 7–2.
A, left-heart failure *(arrow)* with accompanying pulmonary edema. **B,** Kerley B lines *(arrow positioned in lower right lung region* of the same x-ray film).

illary shunting associated with the disorder. Hypoxemia caused by capillary shunting is often refractory to oxygen therapy.

Methods of Decreasing the Hydrostatic Pressure

In an effort to lower the elevated hydrostatic pressure, the physician may order the following:

- Positioning the patient in the Fowler position (sitting up)
- Rotating tourniquets (rarely used today)
- Phlebotomy (rarely used today)

Medications

Morphine Sulfate.—This agent is used to induce venodilation and venous pooling and for psychic sedation.

Diuretic Agents.—Diuretic agents are administered to promote fluid excretion (see Appendix X).

Positive Inotropic Agents.—When heart failure is present, positive inotropic drugs are commonly administered to increase cardiac output (see Appendix IX).

Sympathomimetic Agents.—Sympathomimetic drugs are administered to patients with pulmonary edema if there are accompanying bronchial spasms (see Appendix II).

Albumin.—Albumin is sometimes administered to increase the patient's oncotic pressure in an effort to offset the increased hydrostatic forces of cardiogenic pulmonary edema.

Alcohol (Ethanol, Ethyl Alcohol).—Because alcohol is a specific surface-active agent, it may be aerosolized into the patient's lungs to lower the surface tension of the frothy secretions. This action enhances the mobilization of secretions. Between 5 and 15 mL of a 30% to 50% alcohol solution is generally administered.

SELF-ASSESSMENT QUESTIONS

Multiple Choice
1. In pulmonary edema, fluid first moves into the
    I. Alveoli.
    II. Perivascular interstitial space.
    III. Bronchioles.
    IV. Peribronchial interstitial space.
        a. I only.
        b. II only.
        c. III only.
        d. I and III only.
        e. II and IV only.

2. What is the normal hydrostatic pressure in the pulmonary capillaries?
   a. 5–10 mm Hg.
   b. 10–15 mm Hg.
   c. 15–20 mm Hg.
   d. 20–25 mm Hg.
   e. 25–30 mm Hg.
3. What is the normal oncotic pressure of the blood?
   a. 5–10 mm Hg.
   b. 10–15 mm Hg.
   c. 15–20 mm Hg.
   d. 20–25 mm Hg.
   e. 25–30 mm Hg.
4. Causes of cardiogenic pulmonary edema include
   I. Rapid transfusion of intravenous fluid.
   II. Right ventricular failure.
   III. Mitral valve disease.
   IV. Pulmonary embolus.
   a. III and IV only.
   b. I and II only.
   c. I, II, and III only.
   d. II, III, and IV only.
   e. I, II, III, and IV.
5. Lung compliance is decreased in pulmonary edema because of
   I. Alveolar interstitial edema.
   II. Decreased alveolar surface tension.
   III. Alveolar shrinkage.
   IV. Decreased lymphatic insufficiency.
   a. I only.
   b. II only.
   c. II and III only.
   d. I and III only.
   e. I, III, and IV only.
6. When lung compliance decreases, the patient's
   I. Tidal volume increases.
   II. Respiratory rate decreases.
   III. Tidal volume decreases.
   IV. Respiratory rate increases.
   V. Tidal volume remains the same.
   a. II only.
   b. I and II only.
   c. III and IV only.
   d. II and V only.
   e. IV and V only.
7. As a result of pulmonary edema, the patient's
   I. RV is decreased.
   II. FRC is increased.
   III. VC is increased.
   IV. TLC is increased.
   a. I only.
   b. I and IV only.
   c. II and III only.
   d. III and IV only.
   e. II, III, and IV only.

8. In patients with noncardiogenic pulmonary edema, the pulmonary wedge pressure is typically about
   a. 5–10 mm Hg.
   b. 10–15 mm Hg.
   c. 15–20 mm Hg.
   d. 20–25 mm Hg.
   e. Greater than 25 mm Hg.

True or False

1. Morphine sulfate induces venodilation.   True ____   False ____
2. Patients with pulmonary edema frequently receive 30% to 50% aerosolized alcohol.   True ____   False ____
3. A patient is said to have orthopnea if dyspnea increases when the patient is in the upright position.   True ____   False ____
4. Kerley B lines on chest x-ray films are believed to originate from edematous interlobular septa.   True ____   False ____
5. Hyperproteinemia reduces oncotic pressure.   True ____   False ____

Fill in the Blank

1. An agent used to increase the patient's oncotic pressure to counteract the increased hydrostatic forces associated with cardiogenic pulmonary edema is _____

Answers appear in Appendix XVII.

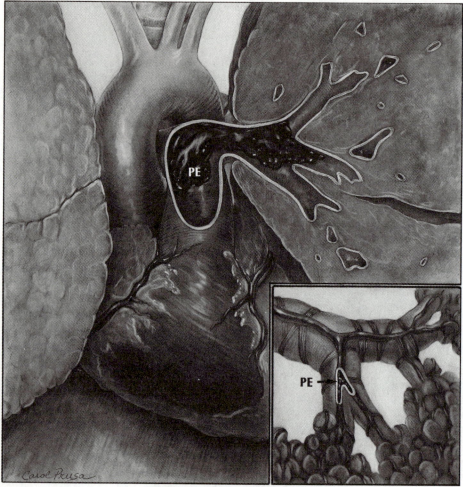

PULMONARY EMBOLISM

FIG 8–1.
Pulmonary embolism *(PE)*.

144

• 8

PULMONARY EMBOLISM

ANATOMIC ALTERATIONS OF THE LUNGS

A pulmonary embolism is a thrombus or other particulate matter that has become dislodged elsewhere in the body and has impacted in the natural filter system of the pulmonary vasculature. Pulmonary embolism is not a primary disease but is a consequence of a disorder outside the pulmonary vascular system.

If the pulmonary embolism significantly disrupts pulmonary blood flow, pulmonary infarction and tissue necrosis will result. Pulmonary embolisms may occur as one large thrombus or as a shower of small thrombi that may or may not interfere with the right heart's ability to perfuse the lungs adequately. When a large embolus detaches from a thrombus and passes through the right heart, it commonly lodges in the bifurcation of the pulmonary artery, where it forms what is known as a saddle embolus (Fig 8–1).

To summarize, the major pathologic or structural changes associated with pulmonary embolism are as follows:

- Blockage of the pulmonary vascular system
- Pulmonary infarction
- Pulmonary tissue necrosis

ETIOLOGY

Although there are many possible sources of pulmonary emboli (e.g., fat, air, amniotic fluid, bone marrow, or tumor fragments), blood clots are by far the most common source.

Most pulmonary emboli originate from a deep vein in the lower part of the body, i.e., the leg and pelvic veins and the inferior vena cava. When a thrombus or a piece of a thrombus breaks loose in a deep vein, the clot is carried through the venous system to the right chambers of the heart and ultimately lodges in the pulmonary arteries or arterioles.

The following are some of the factors predisposing to pulmonary embolisms:

- Venous stasis
  - Prolonged bed rest and/or immobilization
  - Prolonged sitting (e.g., car or plane travel)
  - Congestive heart failure

145

- • Varicose veins
- • Thrombophlebitis
- Trauma
  - • Bone fractures (especially of the pelvis and the long bones of the lower extremities)
  - • Injury to soft tissue
- Postoperative or postpartum states
  - • Extensive hip or abdominal operations
  - • Phlegmasia alba dolens (milk leg)
- Hypercoagulation disorders
  - • Oral contraceptives
  - • Polycythemia
  - • Multiple myeloma
- Others
  - • Obesity
  - • Malignant neoplasms
  - • Pregnancy
  - • Burns

OVERVIEW OF THE CARDIOPULMONARY CLINICAL MANIFESTATIONS ASSOCIATED WITH PULMONARY EMBOLISM

INCREASED RESPIRATORY RATE

There are probably several unique mechanisms working simultaneously to increase the rate of breathing in patients with pulmonary embolism, the major of which follow:

STIMULATION OF PERIPHERAL CHEMORECEPTORS

When an embolus lodges in the pulmonary vascular system, blood flow is reduced or completely absent distal to the obstruction. Consequently, the alveolar ventilation beyond the obstruction is wasted, or dead space, ventilation. That is, there is no carbon dioxide–oxygen exchange. The $\dot{V}/\dot{Q}$ ratio* distal to the pulmonary embolus is high and may even be infinite if there is no perfusion at all (Fig 8–2).

Although portions of the lungs have a high $\dot{V}/\dot{Q}$ ratio at the onset of a pulmonary embolism, this condition is subsequently reversed, and there is a decrease in the $\dot{V}/\dot{Q}$ ratio. In response to the pulmonary embolus, humoral agents such as serotonin and prostaglandin are believed to be released into the pulmonary circulation and cause bronchial constriction. This action in turn leads to a decreased alveolar ventilation relative to alveolar perfusion (decreased $\dot{V}/\dot{Q}$ ratio) and causes a shunt-like effect† and venous admixture‡ (Fig 8–3). Because of the venous admixture, the patient's Pa_{O_2} and Ca_{O_2} decrease. *It should be emphasized that it is not the pulmonary embolism but rather the decreased $\dot{V}/\dot{Q}$ ratio that develops from the pulmonary embolism that actually causes the reduction of the patient's arterial oxygen levels.* As this condition intensifies, the patient's oxygen level may decline to a

*See the section on the ventilation perfusion ratio, page 16.
†See the section on pulmonary shunting, page 18.
‡See the section on venous admixture, page 19.

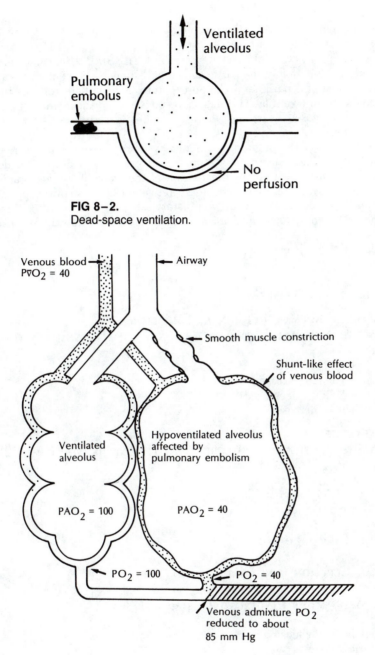

FIG 8–2.
Dead-space ventilation.

FIG 8–3.
Venous admixture in pulmonary embolism.

research purposes may not be combined in one study. As a matter of fact, the integration of these methods is typical in social policy research, where various policy models are studied using different perspectives as well as all kinds of observational and documentary analysis techniques.

Historical/comparative study

The general purpose of a historical/comparative study is to trace the development of specific forms of human social system over sufficiently long periods of time, and to compare those developmental processes across regions, nations, and cultures. This involves the use of historical methods by sociologists, economists, political scientists, and other social scientists. The reason why "historical" always goes with "comparative" is perhaps due to the fact that a comparative study can hardly be accomplished without some far-reaching historical analysis. On the other hand, a historical study would not have the full use to the social scientists if not put in comparative contexts.

Documentary analysis, including the technique of content analysis, has been shown to be the most important approach to a historical/comparative study. By taking advantage of all kinds of documented data from such sources as libraries and archives, government agencies, commercial and non-profit organizations, and private collections, the researcher can gain a view and insight that any other direct data collection strategy may not be able to offer. These, however, depend largely on the credibility and thoroughness of the information recorded in the materials and documents. For the researcher, the way of presenting and interpreting the data, including existing statistics, is equally important. There are probably more pitfalls in a cross-national comparative study than in any other kind of research because of the profound differences between social systems, cultures, and histories. Mistakes can be contained in hasty conclusions due to the unfamiliarity with one or more parties involved.

A multifaceted research design may be the best way to avoid or reduce such mistakes (Chen, 1996). A comparative study often involves site visits in order to get a sense of the realities within different social and cultural systems. Field research including community case studies may also be helpful if permitted by time and other resources. Familiarity with any system other than the researcher's own, however, requires some immersion in that unique social, cultural, and historical context. For this reason, those who have cross-cultural and cross-national life experience are at an advantage in comparative research. This, of

point low enough to stimulate the peripheral chemoreceptors,‡ which in turn initiates an increased ventilatory rate.

REFLEXES FROM THE AORTIC AND CAROTID SINUS BARORECEPTORS

The normal function of the aortic and carotid sinus baroreceptors, located near the aortic and carotid peripheral chemoreceptors, is to initiate reflexes that cause decreased heart and ventilatory rates in response to an elevated systemic blood pressure and increased heart and ventilatory rates in response to a reduced systemic blood pressure.

If obstruction of the pulmonary vascular system is severe, left ventricular output will diminish and cause the systemic blood pressure to drop. The decreased systemic blood pressure reduces the tension of the walls of the aorta and carotid artery, which activates the baroreceptors. Activation of the baroreceptors in turn initiates an increased heart rate and ventilatory rate.

Other pathophysiologic mechanisms may include the following (see page 23):

- Stimulation of the J receptors
- Anxiety

ARTERIAL BLOOD GASES

EARLY STAGES OF PULMONARY EMBOLISM
ACUTE ALVEOLAR HYPERVENTILATION WITH HYPOXEMIA (see page 48)
- Pa_{O_2}: decreased
- Pa_{CO_2}: decreased
- HCO_3^-: decreased
- pH: increased

ADVANCED STAGES OF PULMONARY EMBOLISM
ACUTE VENTILATORY FAILURE WITH HYPOXEMIA (see page 52)
- Pa_{O_2}: decreased
- Pa_{CO_2}: increased
- HCO_3^-: increased
- pH: decreased

CYANOSIS (see page 16)

PLEURAL EFFUSION (see Chapter 12)

CHEST ASSESSMENT FINDINGS (see page 3)

- Crackles/rhonchi/wheezing
- Pleural friction rub

PULMONARY HYPERTENSION

- Cor pulmonale
- Increased central venous pressure (CVP)
- Distended neck veins
- Swollen liver

‡See the section on peripheral chemoreceptors, page 28.

Normally, the pulmonary artery pressure is 25/10 mm Hg, with a mean pulmonary artery pressure of around 15 mm Hg. Most patients with pulmonary embolism, however, have a mean pulmonary artery pressure in excess of 20 mm Hg. Three major mechanisms may contribute to the pulmonary hypertension: (1) decreased cross-sectional area of the pulmonary vascular system due to the emboli, (2) vasoconstriction induced by humoral agents, and (3) vasoconstriction induced by alveolar hypoxia.

Decreased Cross-Sectional Area of the Pulmonary Vascular System Due to the Embolus.—The cross-sectional area of the pulmonary vascular system may decrease significantly if a large embolus becomes lodged in a major artery or if many small emboli become lodged in numerous small pulmonary vessels.

Vasoconstriction Induced by Humoral Agents.—One of the consequences of pulmonary embolism is the release of certain humoral agents, primarily serotonin and prostaglandin. These agents induce smooth muscle constriction of both the tracheobronchial tree and the pulmonary vascular system. Such smooth muscle constriction may further reduce the total cross-sectional area of the pulmonary vascular system and cause the pulmonary artery pressure to rise.

Vasoconstriction Induced by Alveolar Hypoxia.—In response to the humoral agents liberated in pulmonary embolism, the smooth muscles of the tracheobronchial tree constrict and cause the $\dot{V}/\dot{Q}$ ratio* to decrease and the $P_{A_{O_2}}$ to decline. Although the precise mechanism is unclear, when the $P_{A_{O_2}}$ decreases, pulmonary vasoconstriction ensues. This action appears to be a normal compensatory mechanism to offset the shunt produced by the underventilated alveoli. When the number of hypoxic areas becomes significant, however, a generalized pulmonary vasoconstriction may develop and further contribute to the increase in pulmonary blood pressure. When the pulmonary embolism is severe, right-heart strain and cor pulmonale may ensue. Cor pulmonale in turn may lead to an increased CVP, distended neck veins, and a swollen and tender liver.

Systemic Hypotension

When pulmonary hypertension and its related clinical manifestations develop, systemic hypotension is nearly always present. This is due to the decrease in the cross-sectional area of the pulmonary vascular system, which reduces blood flow to the left heart and causes a decrease in left ventricular output and systemic hypotension.

Syncope, Light-headedness, and Confusion

If the left ventricular output and systemic blood pressure decrease substantially, blood flow to the brain may also diminish significantly. This condition may cause periods of light-headedness, confusion, and even syncope.

Increased Heart Rate

The two major mechanisms responsible for the increased heart rate associated with pulmonary embolism are (1) reflexes from the aortic and carotid sinus baroreceptors and (2) stimulation of the pulmonary reflex mechanism.

For a discussion of reflexes from the aortic and carotid sinus baroreceptors, see

---

*See the section on ventilation-perfusion ratio, page 16.

the previous section on increased respiratory rate in this chapter. The increased heart rate may also reflect an indirect response of the heart to hypoxic stimulation of the peripheral chemoreceptors, mainly the carotid bodies.* When the carotid bodies are so stimulated, the patient's ventilatory rate increases. As a result of the increased rate of lung inflation, the pulmonary reflex mechanism is activated; this mechanism triggers tachycardia.†

ABNORMAL ELECTROCARDIOGRAPHIC PATTERNS

- Sinus tachycardia
- Atrial arrhythmias
- Atrial tachycardia
- Atrial flutter
- Atrial fibrillation

In some cases, the obstruction of pulmonary blood flow that is produced by pulmonary emboli leads to abnormal electrocardiographic (ECG) patterns. However, there is no ECG pattern diagnostic of pulmonary embolism. Abnormal patterns merely suggest the possibility. Sinus tachycardia is the most common arrhythmia seen in pulmonary embolism. The sinus tachycardia and atrial arrhythmias sometimes noted in pulmonary embolism are also thought to be indirectly related to the increased right-heart strain and cor pulmonale.

ABNORMAL HEART SOUNDS

- Increased second heart sound (S_2)
- Increased splitting of the second heart sound (S_2)
- Third heart sound (or ventricular gallop)

INCREASED SECOND HEART SOUND (S_2)

Following pulmonary embolization, abnormally high blood pressure develops in the pulmonary artery. This condition causes the pulmonic valve to close more forcefully. As a result, the sound produced by the pulmonic valve (P_2) is often louder than the aortic sound (A_2) is, which causes a louder second heart sound, or S_2.

INCREASED SPLITTING OF THE SECOND HEART SOUND (S_2)

Two major mechanisms either individually or together may contribute to the increased splitting of S_2 sometimes noted in pulmonary embolism: (1) increased pulmonary hypertension and (2) incomplete right bundle-branch block.

In response to the increased pulmonary hypertension associated with pulmonary embolism, the blood pressure in the pulmonic valve area is frequently higher than normal during ventricular contraction. This delays closure of the pulmonic valve and therefore abnormally widens the S_2 split.

The incomplete right bundle-branch block that sometimes accompanies pulmonary embolism may also contribute to the increased splitting of S_2. In an incomplete block, the electrical activity through the right heart is delayed; this delayed activity in turn slows right ventricular contraction. The blood pressure in the pulmonic valve area remains higher than normal and for a longer period of time during right ventricular contraction. As a result, there is delayed closure of the pulmonic valve, which may further widen the S_2 split.

*See the section on peripheral chemoreceptors, page 28.
†See the section on increased heart rate/cardiac output, and blood pressure, page 57.

Third Heart Sound (Ventricular Gallop)

A third heart sound (S_3), or ventricular gallop, is sometimes heard in patients with pulmonary embolism. It occurs early in diastole, about 0.12 to 0.16 seconds after S_2. Although its precise origin is unknown, it is thought that S_3 is created by vibrations during diastole when the rush of blood into the ventricles is abruptly stopped by ventricular walls that have lost some of their elasticity because of hypertrophy.

Thus, when pulmonary embolism causes right-heart strain, or hypertrophy, an S_3, or ventricular gallop, may be noted. An S_3 generated in the right ventricle usually is best heard to the right of the apex close to the lower sternal border and during inspiration.

Other Cardiac Manifestations

Right Ventricular Heave or Lift

As a consequence of the elevated pulmonary blood pressure, right ventricular strain and/or right ventricular hypertrophy often develops. When this occurs, a sustained lift of the chest wall can be felt at the lower left side of the sternum during systole (Fig 8–4). This is because the right ventricle lies directly beneath the sternum.

Cough/Hemoptysis

As a result of the pulmonary hypertension, the pulmonary hydrostatic pressure, normally about 15 mm Hg, often becomes higher than the pulmonary oncotic pressure is (normally about 25 mm Hg). This permits plasma and red blood cells to move across the alveolar-capillary membrane and into alveolar spaces. If this process continues, the subepithelial mechanoreceptors located in the bronchioles, bronchi, and trachea will be stimulated. Such stimulation initiates a cough reflex and the expectoration of blood-tinged sputum.

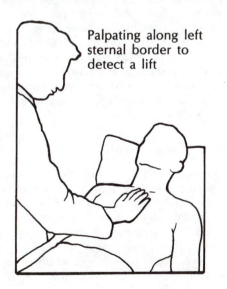

Palpating along left sternal border to detect a lift

FIG 8–4.
A right ventricular lift can sometimes be detected in patients with a pulmonary embolism.

Chest Pain/Decreased Chest Expansion (see page 70)

Chest pain is frequently noted in patients with pulmonary embolism. The origin of the pain is obscure. It may be cardiac or pleural, but it is one of the common, early findings in all forms of pulmonary embolism, even in the absence of obvious cor pulmonale or pleural involvement.

Chest X-Ray Findings

• Increased density
• Hyperradiolucency distal to the embolus
• Dilatation of the pulmonary artery
• Pulmonary edema
• Cor pulmonale
• Pleural effusion

Although there are often no radiographic signs seen in patients with a pulmonary embolus, a density similar to pneumonia with a diffuse border may be seen. There may also be hyperradiolucency distal to the embolus that is caused by decreased vasculature perfusion. Dilatation of the pulmonary artery on the affected side, pulmonary edema (common in a fat embolus), cor pulmonale, and pleural effusion may also be seen.

Abnormal Perfusion Lung Scan vs. Normal Ventilation Scan Findings

An intravenous injection of radiolabeled particles 10 to 50 μm in diameter is useful in determining the presence of pulmonary embolism. Particles labeled with a γ-emitting isotope, usually iodine or technetium, are injected into venous blood. The isotope accompanies the venous blood through the right-heart chambers and on into the pulmonary vascular system. Because blood flow is decreased or absent distal to a pulmonary embolus, fewer radioactive particles are present in this area. This is recorded by an external scintillation camera (Fig 8–5).

Ventilation lung scanning can provide additional information on perfusion defects. The patient breathes a gas mixture containing a small amount of radioactive gas, usually xenon 133. The presence of the xenon is detected by an external scintillation camera during a wash-in or wash-out breathing maneuver. Patients with pulmonary embolism often demonstrate normal ventilation in the region of their perfusion defect (see Fig 8–5).

Abnormal Pulmonary Angiographic Findings

Pulmonary angiography is used to confirm the presence of pulmonary embolism. A catheter is advanced through the right heart and into the pulmonary artery. A radiopaque dye is then rapidly injected into the pulmonary artery while serial roentgenograms are taken. Pulmonary embolism is confirmed by abnormal filling within the artery or a cutoff of the artery. A dark area appears on the angiogram distal to the embolization since the radiopaque material is prevented from flowing past the obstruction (Fig 8–6). The procedure generally poses no risk to the patient unless there is severe pulmonary hypertension (mean pulmonary artery pressure >45 mm Hg) or the patient is in shock.

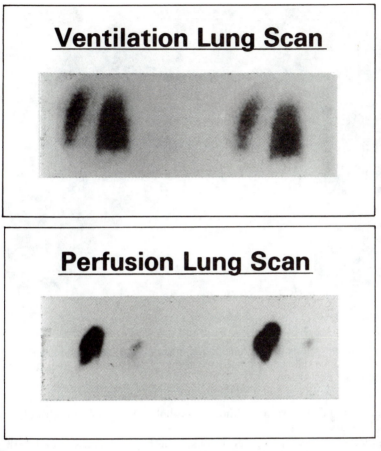

FIG 8–5.
Abnormal perfusion scan and normal ventilation scan findings are commonly seen in patients with severe pulmonary embolism.

GENERAL MANAGEMENT OF PULMONARY EMBOLISM

Preventive Measures

Preventive measures should be initiated in patients who are predisposed to pulmonary embolism. Low doses of subcutaneous heparin have been proved extremely helpful in these patients. Tight-fitting elastic stockings have been helpful in patients prone to thrombosis of the leg veins.

Management of Pulmonary Embolism

Heparin, administered intravenously, is the primary anticoagulant used to treat patients with pulmonary embolism. Warfarin and dicumarol are the most commonly used oral anticoagulants. These agents are used primarily for the prevention

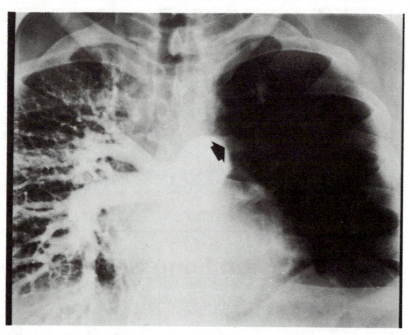

FIG 8–6.
Abnormal pulmonary angiogram. Radiopaque material injected into the blood is prevented from flowing past the pulmonary embolism *(arrow)*. This causes the angiogram to appear dark distal to the obstruction.

of any additional or recurrent pulmonary emboli. They do nothing to eliminate existing pulmonary emboli.

Supplemental oxygen is given to offset the hypoxemia associated with pulmonary embolization. Cardiotonic drugs are sometimes employed to reduce right-heart strain, and ECG monitoring is used to detect heart arrhythmias.

Thrombolytic Agents

Urokinase and streptokinase, two fibrinolytic agents, have been proved beneficial in treating pulmonary embolism. These thrombolytic agents are sometimes used along with heparin. Because of the excessive risk of bleeding, however, the use of fibrinolytic agents in treating pulmonary embolism has been limited.

Pulmonary Embolectomy

Surgical removal of blood clots from the pulmonary circulation is generally a last resort in treating pulmonary embolism because of the excessive mortality of the procedure and because of the availability of fibrinolytic agents to treat pulmonary embolism.

SELF-ASSESSMENT QUESTIONS

Multiple Choice

1. Most pulmonary emboli originate from the
   a. Lungs.
   b. Right heart.
   c. Leg and pelvic veins.
   d. Left heart.
   e. Pulmonary veins.

2. The aortic and carotid sinus baroreceptors initiate the following in response to a decreased systemic blood pressure:
   I. Increased heart rate.
   II. Increased ventilatory rate.
   III. Decreased heart rate.
   IV. Decreased ventilatory rate.
   V. Ventilatory rate is not affected by the aortic and carotid sinus baroreceptors.
   a. I and IV only.
   b. II and III only.
   c. III and IV only.
   d. I and II only.
   e. V only.

3. What is the normal mean pulmonary artery pressure?
   a. 5 mm Hg.
   b. 10 mm Hg.
   c. 15 mm Hg.
   d. 20 mm Hg.
   e. 25 mm Hg.

4. Pulmonary hypertension develops in pulmonary embolism because of
   I. Increased cross-sectional area of the pulmonary vascular system.
   II. Vasoconstriction due to humoral agent release.
   III. Vasoconstriction induced by decreased arterial oxygen pressure (Pa_{O_2}).
   IV. Vasoconstriction induced by decreased alveolar oxygen pressure (PA_{O_2}).
   a. I and III only.
   b. II and III only.
   c. I, II, and III only.
   d. II, III, and IV only.
   e. II and IV only.

5. S_1 is associated with the closure of the
   I. Tricuspid valve.
   II. Pulmonic valve.
   III. Mitral valve.
   IV. Semilunar valve.
   a. I only.
   b. IV only.
   c. I and III only.
   d. III and IV only.
   e. II, III, and IV only.

6. S_2 is sometimes louder in pulmonary embolism because of a more forceful closure of the
   a. Tricuspid valve.
   b. Pulmonic valve.

    c. Mitral valve.

    d. Bicuspid valve.

7. When humoral agents such as serotonin are released into the pulmonary circulation,

   I. The bronchial smooth muscles dilate.

   II. The $\dot{V}/\dot{Q}$ ratio decreases.

   III. The bronchial smooth muscles constrict.

   IV. The $\dot{V}/\dot{Q}$ ratio increases

    a. I only.

    b. II only.

    c. IV only.

    d. II and III only.

    e. I and IV only.

8. Which of the following is a thrombolytic agent?

   I. Urokinase.

   II. Heparin.

   III. Warfarin.

   IV. Streptokinase.

    a. I only.

    b. IV only.

    c. II and III only.

    d. I and IV only.

    e. I, II, III, and IV.

9. What is/are the most prominent source of pulmonary emboli?

    a. Fat.

    b. Blood clots.

    c. Bone marrow.

    d. Air.

    e. Malignant neoplasms.

10. Which of the following is the most common arrhythmia seen in pulmonary embolism?

    a. Sinus tachycardia.

    b. Atrial flutter.

    c. Left bundle-branch block.

    d. Incomplete right bundle-branch block.

    e. Complete right bundle-branch block.

Answers appear in Appendix XVII.

course, does not mean that personal experiences and haphazard observations may replace systematic training and structured research effort. However, it is apparent that a superficial understanding, or simply playing with the numbers, is not enough. Here a qualitative understanding derived from all sources of information is crucial in making a pertinent comparison.

Evaluation research

Evaluation is a most commonly seen intellectual and social activity in our daily life. Its becoming a most popular form of social research, however, is a recent trend tied with the increasingly recognized need for social program evaluation (Royse & Thyer, 1996). Evaluation research is concerned with the impact, or effectiveness, and the efficiency of the intervention embodied in a social program. This type of research helps to formulate, monitor, as well as evaluate social programs. In real terms, evaluation has increasingly become an inherent part of new program requirements. Available funding for program evaluation has also attracted enormous attention from social scientists who are interested in applied research.

Since evaluation is so closely tied to the program itself, the situation of program design and implementation will constantly impact on evaluation research. For instance, the objectives and independent and dependent variables of evaluation research are often directly derived from the published and unpublished documents of a program in terms of its goals, interventions, and outcomes. However, anyone who has studied public policy making and implementation should know that the goals of a program may change, the interventions can be very vague, and the expectations on its outcomes may be contradictory with one another. All these would pose serious challenges to evaluation research. As a matter of fact, one of the important functions of evaluation research is to help overcome some of the major problems in program design and implementation.

Evaluation research usually adopts a longitudinal design. The basic logic used for most evaluation research projects is what underlies social experimentation. Nevertheless, the classical experimental model is often difficult to apply to the real research situation, especially in terms of the randomization of the assignment of subjects to experimental and control groups. In such cases, evaluation research would call for "quasi-experimental" designs. These include the use of non-randomly assigned (nonequivalent but comparable) control groups and time-series analysis.

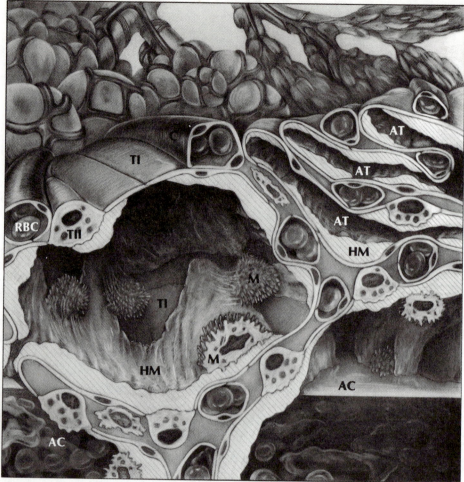

ADULT RESPIRATORY DISTRESS SYNDROME

FIG 9–1.
Adult respiratory distress syndrome. *RBC* = red blood cell; *TI* = type I cell; *TII* = type II cell; *C* = capillaries; *AT* = atelectasis; *HM* = hyaline membrane; *M* = macrophages; *AC* = alveolar consolidation.

ADULT RESPIRATORY DISTRESS SYNDROME

ANATOMIC ALTERATIONS OF THE LUNGS

The lungs of patients affected by adult respiratory distress syndrome (ARDS) undergo similar anatomic changes, regardless of the etiology of the disease. In response to injury, the pulmonary capillaries become engorged, and the permeability of the alveolar-capillary membrane increases. Interstitial and intra-alveolar edema and hemorrhage ensue, as well as scattered areas of hemorrhagic alveolar consolidation. These processes result in a decrease in alveolar surfactant and in alveolar collapse, or atelectasis.

As the disease progresses, the intra-alveolar walls become lined with a thick, ripply hyaline membrane identical to the hyaline membrane seen in the newborn with infant respiratory distress syndrome (hyaline membrane disease). The membrane contains fibrin and cellular debris. In prolonged cases there is hyperplasia and swelling of the type II cells. Fibrin and exudate develop and lead to intra-alveolar fibrosis.

In gross appearance, the lungs of ARDS victims are heavy and "red," "beefy," or "liverlike" in appearance. The anatomic alterations that develop in ARDS create a restrictive lung disorder (Fig 9–1).

To summarize, the major pathologic or structural changes associated with ARDS are as follows:

- Interstitial and intra-alveolar edema and hemorrhage
- Alveolar consolidation
- Intra-alveolar hyaline membrane
- Pulmonary surfactant deficiency or abnormality
- Atelectasis

Historically, ARDS was referred to as "shock lung syndrome" when the disease was first identified in combat casualties during World War II. Since that time, the disease has appeared in the medical literature under many different names, all based on the etiology believed to be responsible for the disease. In 1967, the disease was first described as a specific entity, and the term *adult respiratory distress syndrome* was suggested. This term is predominantly used today. In alphabetical order, some of the names that have appeared in the medical journals to identify ARDS are as follows:

- Acute alveolar failure
- Adult hyaline membrane disease
- Capillary leak syndrome
- Congestion atelectasis
- Da Nang lung (because of the high incidence of ARDS associated with casualties in the Viet Nam War)
- Hemorrhagic pulmonary edema
- Noncardiac pulmonary edema
- Oxygen pneumonitis
- Oxygen toxicity
- Postnontraumatic pulmonary insufficiency
- Postperfusion lung
- Postpump lung
- Posttraumatic pulmonary insufficiency
- Shock lung syndrome
- Stiff lung syndrome
- Wet lung
- White lung syndrome

ETIOLOGY

There appears to be a multitude of etiologic factors that may produce ARDS. In alphabetical order are some of the better-known causes of ARDS:

- Aspiration (e.g., of gastric contents or of water in near-drowning episodes)
- Central nervous system (CNS) disease (particularly when complicated by increased intracranial pressure)
- Cardiopulmonary bypass (especially when the surgical procedure is prolonged)
- Congestive heart failure (leads to increased alveolar fluid leakage)
- Disseminated intravascular coagulation (seen in patients with shock and is a paradox of simultaneous clotting and bleeding to produce microthrombi in the lungs)
- Drug overdose (e.g., heroin, barbiturates, morphine, methadone)
- Fat or air emboli (the fat emboli act as a source of harmful vasoactive material such as fatty acids and serotonin)
- Fluid overload (promotes alveolar fluid leakage)
- Infections (bacterial, viral, fungal, parasitic, mycoplasmal)
- Inhalation of toxins and irritants (e.g., chlorine gas, nitrogen dioxide, smoke, ozone; oxygen may also be included in this section)
- Immunologic reaction (e.g., allergic alveolar reaction to inhaled material or Goodpasture's syndrome)
- Massive blood transfusion (in stored blood, the quantity of aggregated white blood cells [WBCs], red blood cells [RBCs], platelets, and fibrin increases; these blood components in turn may occlude or damage small blood vessels)
- Nonthoracic trauma
- Oxygen toxicity (e.g., when patients are treated with an excessive $F_{I_{O_2}}$—usually over 60%—for a prolonged period of time)

- Pulmonary ischemia (due to shock and hypoperfusion; may cause tissue necrosis, vascular damage, and capillary leak)
- Radiation-induced lung injury
- Shock (e.g., hypovolemia)
- Systemic reactions to processes initiated outside the lungs (e.g., reactions caused by hemorrhagic pancreatitis, burns, complicated abdominal surgery, septicemia)
- Thoracic trauma (i.e., direct contusion to the lungs)
- Uremia

OVERVIEW OF THE CARDIOPULMONARY CLINICAL MANIFESTATIONS ASSOCIATED WITH ADULT RESPIRATORY DISTRESS SYNDROME

INCREASED RESPIRATORY RATE

Several pathophysiologic mechanisms operating simultaneously may lead to an increased ventilatory rate. These are (see page 23):

- Stimulation of peripheral chemoreceptors
- Decreased lung compliance/increased work of breathing relationship
- Stimulation of the J receptors
- Anxiety

PULMONARY FUNCTION STUDIES

LUNG VOLUME AND CAPACITY FINDINGS (see page 37)
- Decreased VC
- Decreased RV
- Decreased FRC
- Decreased TLC
- Decreased V_T

INCREASED HEART RATE, CARDIAC OUTPUT, AND BLOOD PRESSURE (see page 57)

ARTERIAL BLOOD GASES

EARLY STAGES OF ARDS
ACUTE ALVEOLAR HYPERVENTILATION WITH HYPOXEMIA (see page 48)
- Pa_{O_2}: decreased
- Pa_{CO_2}: decreased
- HCO_3^-: decreased
- pH: increased

ADVANCED STAGES OF ARDS
ACUTE VENTILATORY FAILURE WITH HYPOXEMIA (see page 52)
- Pa_{O_2}: decreased
- Pa_{CO_2}: increased
- HCO_3^-: increased
- pH: decreased

CYANOSIS (see page 16)

SUBSTERNAL INTERCOSTAL RETRACTIONS (see page 72)

CHEST ASSESSMENT FINDINGS (see page 3)

- Dull percussion note
- Bronchial breath sounds

CHEST X-RAY FINDINGS

INCREASED OPACITY

The structural changes that develop in ARDS increase the density of the lungs. The increase in lung density resists x-ray penetration and is revealed on x-ray films as increased opacity (i.e., whiter in appearance). Thus, the more severe the ARDS is, the denser the lungs become, and the whiter the x-ray film will be (see Fig 9–2).

GENERAL MANAGEMENT OF ARDS

Hyperinflation Techniques

Hyperinflation measures are commonly ordered to offset the alveolar consolidation and atelectasis associated with ARDS (see Appendix XII).

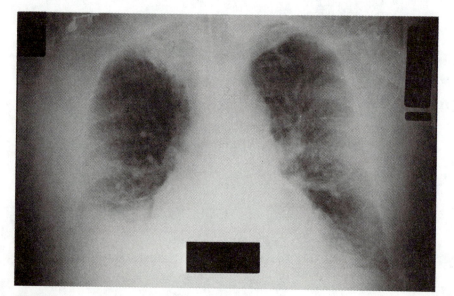

FIG 9–2.
Chest x-ray of patient with severe ARDS.

Medications

Diuretic Agents.—Diuretic agents are frequently ordered for patients with ARDS to counteract the fluid overload (see Appendix X).

Corticosteroids.—Although the exact mode of action of corticosteroids is not known, they have been shown to be effective in treating patients with ARDS (see Appendix V). The corticosteroids are used to suppress inflammation and edema.

Antibiotic Agents.—Antibiotics are frequently administered in an effort to prevent secondary bacterial infection (see Appendix VIII).

Supplemental Oxygen

Because of the hypoxemia associated with ARDS, supplemental oxygen may be required. It should be noted, however, that the hypoxemia that develops in ARDS is most commonly caused by the alveolar consolidation, atelectasis, and capillary shunting associated with the disorder. Hypoxemia caused by capillary shunting is often refractory to oxygen therapy.

SELF-ASSESSMENT QUESTIONS

Multiple Choice
1. In response to injury, the lungs of an ARDS patient undergo these changes:
    I. Atelectasis.
    II. Decreased alveolar-capillary membrane permeability.
    III. Interstitial and intra-alveolar edema.
    IV. Hemorrhagic alveolar consolidation.
        a. I and III only.
        b. II and IV only.
        c. I, II, and IV only.
        d. I, III, and IV only.
        e. I, II, III, and IV.
2. Historically, ARDS was first referred to as
        a. Oxygen toxicity.
        b. Shock lung syndrome.
        c. Adult hyaline membrane disease.
        d. Congestion atelectasis.
        e. White lung.
3. The generic name of Lasix is
        a. Furosemide.
        b. Spironolactone.
        c. Aldactone.
        d. Thiazide.
        e. Hydrochlorothiazide.
4. During the early stages of ARDS, the patient commonly demonstrates which arterial blood gas values?
    I. Decreased pH.
    II. Increased Pa_{CO_2}.
    III. Decreased HCO_3^-

    IV. Normal Pa_{O_2}.
       a. II only.
       b. III only.
       c. II and III only.
       d. III and IV only.
       e. I and II only.

True or False

1. The hyaline membrane that develops in ARDS is identical to the hyaline membrane seen in the newborn with infant respiratory distress syndrome.   True _____   False _____
2. The lung compliance of patients with ARDS is very high.   True _____   False _____
3. The J receptors are located in the terminal bronchioles.   True _____   False _____
4. The RV is increased in patients with ARDS.   True _____   False _____
5. Chest x-ray findings in ARDS reveal a decreased opacity.   True _____   False _____

Answers appear in Appendix XVII.

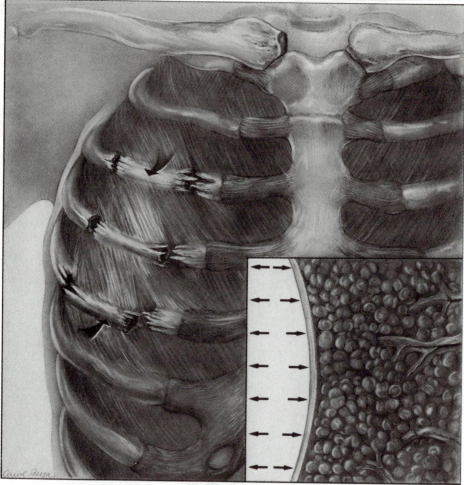

FLAIL CHEST

FIG 10–1.
Flail chest. *Inset:* alveoli collapsing as a result of the flail chest. Double fractures of at least three or more adjacent ribs *(arrows).*

FLAIL CHEST

ANATOMIC ALTERATIONS OF THE LUNGS

A flail chest is the result of double fractures of at least three or more adjacent ribs, which causes the thoracic cage to become unstable (Fig 10–1). The affected ribs cave in (flail) during inspiration as a result of the subatmospheric intrapleural pressure. This compresses and restricts the underlying lung area and promotes atelectasis and lung collapse. In severe cases there may also be contusion of the lung under the fractured ribs.

To summarize, the major pathologic or structural changes associated with flail chest are as follows:

- Double fracture of multiple adjacent ribs
- Rib instability
- Lung restriction
- Atelectasis
- Lung collapse

ETIOLOGY

A crushing injury to the chest is usually the cause of a flail chest. Such trauma may result from the following:

- Direct compression by a heavy object
- Automobile accident
- Industrial accident

OVERVIEW OF THE CARDIOPULMONARY CLINICAL MANIFESTATIONS ASSOCIATED WITH FLAIL CHEST

INCREASED RESPIRATORY RATE

Several pathophysiologic mechanisms operating simultaneously may lead to an increased ventilatory rate. These are:

STIMULATION OF PERIPHERAL CHEMORECEPTORS

As a result of the paradoxical movement of the chest wall, the lung area directly beneath the broken ribs is compressed during inspiration and is pushed out-

The application of the conventional experimental model including such "quasi" designs, however, is not the only approach to evaluation research. In real terms, the traditional model has been criticized by philosophers of science and theorists of methodology and is regarded as failing to address the issue of conflicting interests of various stakeholders in politicized research settings. Alternative models of evaluation have therefore been developed, with the explosive development of qualitative evaluation methods over last two decades. From the point of view of methodology advancement, this renders an excellent opportunity to triangulate your research design for the purpose of a more adequate assessment and evaluation of a program. For the task of needs assessment (now an integral and important part of formative evaluation), for example, the technique of focus groups can be used to supplement standardized questionnaire surveys (Krueger, 1994).

Within the family of quantitative methods and approaches, there are also ways for triangulation. In the California Work Pays Demonstration Project mentioned earlier, for example, data are not only extracted monthly from county administrative records but also obtained from multi-wave questionnaire surveys. Generally speaking, a real evaluation project tends to collect data from multiple sources and use multiple approaches to serve the same research purpose.

Making the most out of a focal method

In the above we were concerned with the use of multiple methods to serve the same research purpose. In this section let us consider how a method can be used in different research situations and serve various research objectives.

Questionnaire survey

Unlike physical science where complex and expensive equipment may be necessary for conducting research, social science studies oftentimes use only paper-and-pencil instruments for data collection. The most important instrument is a standardized questionnaire. The questionnaire can be administered through face-to-face or telephone interview, or sent out for self-administration and collected by mail. Data collection by means of the standardized questionnaire is now so widely used that it has become a central element in survey research. Sometimes people would simply call the administration of a questionnaire, or

ward through the flail area during expiration. This abnormal chest and lung movement causes air to be shunted from one lung to another during a ventilatory cycle.

When the lung on the affected side is compressed during inspiration, gas moves into the lung on the unaffected side. During expiration, however, air from the unaffected lung moves into the affected lung. The shunting of air from one lung to another is known as *pendelluft* (Fig 10–2). In consequence of the pendelluft, the patient rebreathes dead-space gas and hypoventilates. In addition to the hypoventilation produced by the pendelluft, alveolar ventilation may also be decreased by the lung compression and atelectasis associated with an unstable chest.

As a result of the pendelluft, lung compression, and atelectasis, the $\dot{V}/\dot{Q}$* ratio decreases. This leads to intrapulmonary shunting† and venous admixture‡ (Fig 10–3). Because of the venous admixture, the patient's Pao_2 and CaO_2 decrease. As this condition intensifies, the patient's oxygen level may decline to a point low enough to stimulate the peripheral chemoreceptors, which, in turn, initiate an increased ventilatory rate.

OTHER POSSIBLE MECHANISMS (see page 23)
- Decreased lung compliance/increased work of breathing relationship
- Activation of the deflation reflex
- Activation of the irritant receptors
- Stimulation of the J receptors
- Pain/anxiety

PULMONARY FUNCTION STUDIES

LUNG VOLUME AND CAPACITY FINDINGS (see page 37)
- Decreased VC
- Decreased RV
- Decreased FRC
- Decreased TLC
- Decreased V_T

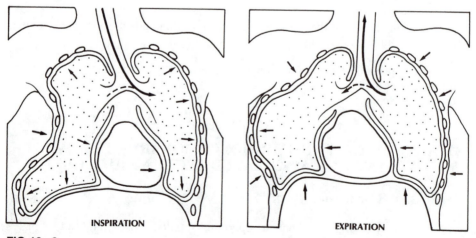

FIG 10–2.
Lateral flail chest with accompanying Pendelluft.

*See the section on ventilation-perfusion ratio, page 16.
†See the section on pulmonary shunting, page 18.
‡See the section on venous admixture, page 19.

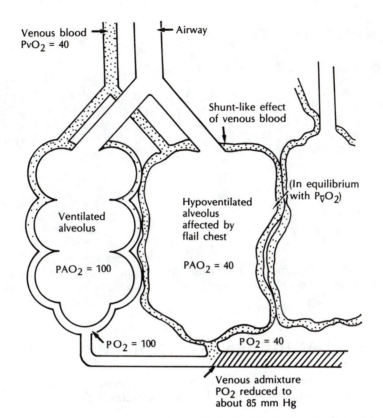

Venous blood
$PvO_2 = 40$

Airway

Shunt-like effect
of venous blood

(In equilibrium
with $P_{\bar{v}}O_2$)

Ventilated
alveolus

$PAO_2 = 100$

Hypoventilated
alveolus
affected by
flail chest

$PAO_2 = 40$

$PO_2 = 100$

$PO_2 = 40$

Venous admixture
PO_2 reduced to
about 85 mm Hg

FIG 10–3.
Venous admixture in flail chest.

INCREASED HEART RATE, CARDIAC OUTPUT, AND BLOOD PRESSURE (see page 57)

INCREASED CENTRAL VENOUS PRESSURE/DECREASED SYSTEMIC BLOOD PRESSURE (see page 57)

ARTERIAL BLOOD GASES

EARLY STAGES OF FLAIL CHEST
ACUTE ALVEOLAR HYPERVENTILATION WITH HYPOXEMIA (see page 48)
- Pa_{O_2}: decreased
- Pa_{CO_2}: decreased
- HCO_3^-: decreased
- pH: increased

ADVANCED STAGES OF FLAIL CHESTS
ACUTE VENTILATORY FAILURE WITH HYPOXEMIA (see page 52)
- Pa_{O_2}: decreased
- Pa_{CO_2}: increased
- HCO_3^-: increased
- pH: decreased

CYANOSIS (see page 16)

PARADOXICAL MOVEMENT OF THE CHEST WALL

When double fractures exist in at least three or more adjacent ribs, a paradoxical movement of the chest wall is seen, that is, during inspiration, the fractured ribs are pushed inward by the atmospheric pressure surrounding the chest. During expiration, the flail area bulges outward when the intrapleural pressure becomes greater than the atomospheric pressure.

CHEST X-RAY FINDINGS

• Increased opacity
• Rib fractures

Because of the lung compression and atelectasis associated with a flail chest, the density of the lungs increases. The increase in lung density is revealed on x-ray films as an increased opacity (i.e., whiter in appearance). X-ray films will also show the rib fractures (Fig 10–4).

GENERAL MANAGEMENT OF FLAIL CHEST

In mild cases, medication for pain and routine bronchial hygiene may be all that is needed. In more severe cases, however, stabilization of the chest is usually

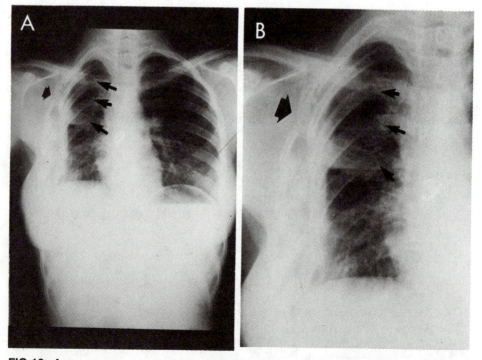

FIG 10–4.
A, chest x-ray film of a 20-year-old female with a severe right-sided flail chest. **B,** close-up of the same x-ray film.

required to allow bone healing and to prevent atelectasis. Today, controlled volume ventilation, sometimes accompanied by positive end-expiratory pressure (PEEP), is commonly used to stabilize a flail chest. Generally, mechanical ventilation for 5 to 10 days is an adequate time for bone healing.

Supplemental Oxygen

Because of the hypoxemia associated with a flail chest, supplemental oxygen may be required. It should be noted, however, that the hypoxemia that develops in a flail chest is most commonly caused by the alveolar atelectasis and capillary shunting associated with the disorder. Hypoxemia caused by capillary shunting is often refractory to oxygen therapy.

SELF-ASSESSMENT QUESTIONS

Multiple Choice
1. When the deflation reflex is activated,
    I. The lungs deflate.
    II. The expiratory time increases.
    III. The ventilatory rate increases.
    IV. The Hering-Breuer inflation reflex is activated.
        a. I only.
        b. II only.
        c. III only.
        d. III and IV only.
        e. I, III, and IV only.
2. When a patient has a severe flail chest,
    I. Venous return increases.
    II. Cardiac output decreases.
    III. Systemic blood pressure increases.
    IV. Central venous pressure increases.
        a. I only.
        b. III only.
        c. III and IV only.
        d. II and IV only.
        e. I, III, and IV only.
3. A flail chest consists of a double fracture of at least
        a. Two adjacent ribs.
        b. Three adjacent ribs.
        c. Four adjacent ribs.
        d. Five adjacent ribs.
        e. Six adjacent ribs.
4. During the advanced stages of a severe flail chest, the patient commonly demonstrates the following arterial blood gas finding:
    I. Decreased Pa_{O_2}.
    II. Decreased Pa_{CO_2}.
    III. Increased HCO_3^-
    IV. Increased pH.
        a. I and II only.
        b. II and III only.
        c. III and IV only.

    d. I and III only.
    e. I, II, and IV only.
5. When the carotid bodies are stimulated, a signal is sent to the medulla by way of cranial nerve
    a. VI.
    b. VII.
    c. VIII.
    d. IX.
    e. X.
6. As a consequence of a severe flail chest, the
    I. RV increases.
    II. VT decreases.
    III. VC increases.
    IV. FRC decreases.
    a. IV only.
    b. I and III only.
    c. II and IV only.
    d. II, III, and IV only.
    e. I, II, III, and IV.
7. When mechanical ventilation is used to stabilize a flail chest, how much time is generally needed for bone healing to occur?
    a. 5–10 days.
    b. 10–15 days.
    c. 15–20 days.
    d. 20–25 days.
    e. 25–30 days.

True or False

1. The shunting of air from one lung to another is known as pendelluft.   True _____   False _____
2. The fractured ribs of a severe flail chest commonly move outward during expiration.   True _____   False _____
3. In pendelluft, lung compression and atelectasis cause the $\dot{V}/\dot{Q}$ ratio to increase.   True _____   False _____
4. The irritant receptors are also known as the subepithelial mechanoreceptors.   True _____   False _____
5. During the advanced stages of a severe flail chest, the increased HCO_3^- level in the arterial blood gases is secondary to the increased Pa_{CO_2}.   True _____   False _____

Answers appear in Appendix XVII.

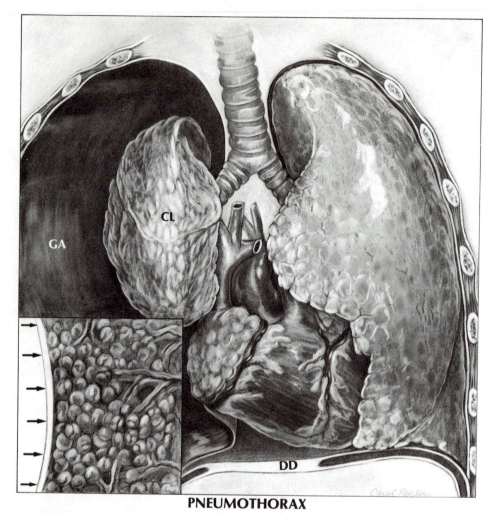

PNEUMOTHORAX

FIG 11–1.
Right-sided pneumothorax. *GA* = gas accumulation; *DD* = depressed diaphragm; *CL* = collapsed lung. *Inset:* alveoli collapsing as a result of pneumothorax.

• 11

PNEUMOTHORAX

ANATOMIC ALTERATIONS OF THE LUNGS

A pneumothorax exists when gas accumulates in the pleural space (Fig 11–1). When gas enters the pleural space, the visceral and parietal pleura separate. This enhances the natural tendency of the lungs to recoil, or collapse, and the natural tendency of the chest wall to move outward, or expand. As the lungs collapse, the alveoli are compressed, and atelectasis ensues. In severe cases, the great veins may be compressed and cause the venous return to diminish.

To summarize, the major pathologic or structural changes associated with a pneumothorax are as follows:

- Lung collapse
- Atelectasis
- Chest wall expansion
- Compression of the great veins and decreased venous return

ETIOLOGY

There are three ways in which gas can gain entrance to the pleural space:

- From the lungs through a perforation of the visceral pleura
- From the surrounding atmosphere through a perforation of the chest wall and parietal pleura or, rarely, through an esophageal fistula or from a perforated abdominal viscus
- From gas-forming microorganisms in an empyema in the pleural space

A pneumothorax may be classified as either closed or open according to how gas gains entrance to the pleural space. In a *closed pneumothorax* gas in the pleural space is not in direct contact with the atmosphere. An *open pneumothorax*, on the other hand, implies that the pleural space is in direct contact with the atmosphere and that gas can move freely in and out. A pneumothorax in which the intrapleural pressure exceeds the intra-alveolar (or atmospheric) pressure is known as a tension pneumothorax. Some etiologic forms of pneumothorax are as follows:

- Traumatic pneumothorax
- Spontaneous pneumothorax
- Iatrogenic pneumothorax

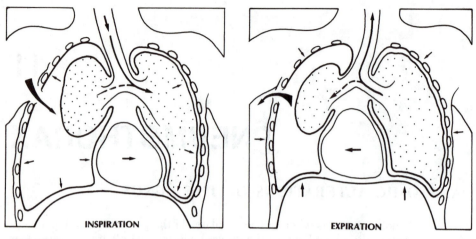

FIG 11–2.
Sucking chest wound with accompanying pendelluft.

Traumatic Pneumothorax

Penetrating wounds to the chest wall from a knife, bullet, or an impaling object in an automobile or industrial accident are common causes of a traumatic pneumothorax. When this type of trauma occurs, the pleural space is in direct contact with the atmosphere, and gas can move in and out of the pleural cavity. This condition is known as a sucking chest wound and is classified as an open pneumothorax (Fig 11–2).

A piercing chest wound may also result in a valvular pneumothorax. In this form of pneumothorax gas enters the pleural space during inspiration but cannot leave during expiration since the chest wall acts as a check valve. This condition may cause the intrapleural pressure to exceed the atmospheric pressure in the affected area. Technically, this form of pneumothorax is classified as a tension pneumothorax (Fig 11–3).

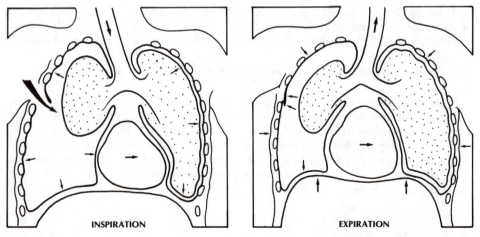

FIG 11–3.
Valvular pneumothorax produced by a chest wall wound.

When a crushing chest injury occurs, the pleural space may not be in direct contact with the atmosphere, but the sharp end of a fractured rib may pierce or tear the visceral pleura. This may permit gas to leak into the pleural space from the lungs. Technically, this form of pneumothorax is classified as a closed pneumothorax.

Spontaneous Pneumothorax

When a pneumothorax occurs suddenly and without any obvious underlying cause, it is referred to as a spontaneous pneumothorax. A spontaneous pneumothorax is often secondary to certain underlying pathologic processes such as pneumonia, tuberculosis, and chronic obstructive pulmonary disease. A spontaneous pneumothorax is sometimes caused by the rupture of a small bleb or bulla on the surface of the lung. This type of pneumothorax often occurs in tall persons between the ages of 15 and 35 years. This may be due to the high negative pressure and mechanical stresses that take place in the upper zone of the upright lung.

A spontaneous pneumothorax may also behave as a valvular pneumothorax. Air from the lung parenchyma may enter the pleural space via a tear in the visceral pleura during inspiration but is unable to leave during expiration since the visceral tear functions as a check valve (Fig 11–4). This condition may cause the intrapleural pressure to exceed the intra-alveolar pressure. Technically, this form of pneumothorax is classified as both a closed and a tension pneumothorax.

Iatrogenic Pneumothorax

An iatrogenic pneumothorax sometimes occurs during specific diagnostic or therapeutic procedures. For example, a pleural or liver biopsy may cause a pneumothorax. Thoracentesis, intercostal nerve block, cannulation of a subclavian vein, and tracheostomy are possible causes of an iatrogenic pneumothorax. An iatrogenic pneumothorax is always a hazard during positive-pressure mechanical ventilation.

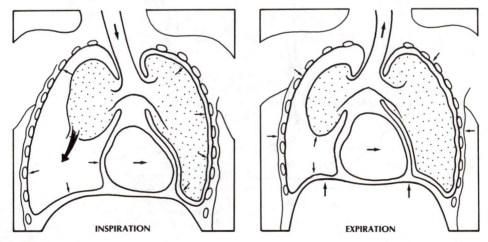

INSPIRATION   EXPIRATION

FIG 11–4.
Valvular pneumothorax produced by a rupture in the visceral pleura.

even a questionnaire itself, a survey.

A survey using a standardized questionnaire is often put on a par with other tools of social science research such as a social experiment. Questionnaire surveys, nevertheless, can be used in both cross-sectional studies ("surveys") and experiments (or generally longitudinal studies). The term "survey research" virtually refers to all kinds of research activities centered on the selection of the respondents and the administration of the questionnaires. In such a sense, survey research methods are not just concerned with a single mode of research but provide many useful techniques that can be applied to different research programs.

Case study

A questionnaire survey can be applied to the study of both large and small samples. No matter what the sample size is, the limitation of a standardized questionnaire survey is in that it can hardly offer a full sense of what has been happening to the subjects in their everyday settings. A case study, on the other hand, focuses on only one or a few cases, and the essence of this technique is that it goes far beyond a questionnaire survey and digs into the details of relevant aspects. The inquiry is usually much more time-consuming, intensive, and focused. Here a "case" can be taken for different units of analysis. It can be an individual, a family or another kind of social group, a formal organization, a local community, a nation, or a national welfare system. The classic case study tended to refer a case to an individual. Yet there was also tremendous effort in community study, as well as case studies using other units of analysis.

Although case study research, either a single-case design or a multiple-case design, may adopt such an analytic strategy as time-series analysis, it is usually considered as only a supplementary approach to social inquiry. Yet it is argued that case study research may directly lead to theoretical generalization, as is commonly seen in natural science (Yin, 1994). In certain social, political, and cultural settings, such as China before "open-door" when a "unification" requirement made all of its parts look alike (Chen, 1996), a special kind of case study research, called "typical example" study, has been a major form of social investigation. Generally speaking, case study research can be used in conjunction with standardized questionnaire surveys in both cross-sectional and longitudinal studies. It can play an important part in different modes of research, including historical/comparative study and evaluation research.

OVERVIEW OF THE CARDIOPULMONARY CLINICAL MANIFESTATIONS ASSOCIATED WITH PNEUMOTHORAX

INCREASED RESPIRATORY RATE

Several pathophysiologic mechanisms operating simultaneously may lead to an increased ventilatory rate. These are:

STIMULATION OF PERIPHERAL CHEMORECEPTORS

As gas moves into the pleural space, the visceral and parietal pleura separate, and the lung on the affected side begins to collapse. As the lung collapses, atelectasis develops, and alveolar ventilation decreases.

If the patient has a pneumothorax due to a sucking chest wound, an additional mechanism may also promote hypoventilation. That is, when a patient with this type of pneumothorax inhales, the intrapleural pressure on the unaffected side decreases. As a result, the mediastinum often moves to the unaffected side, where the pressure is lower, and compresses the normal lung. The intrapleural pressure on the affected side may also decrease, and some air may enter through the chest wound and further shift the mediastinum toward the normal lung. During expiration, the intrapleural pressure on the affected side rises above atmospheric pres-

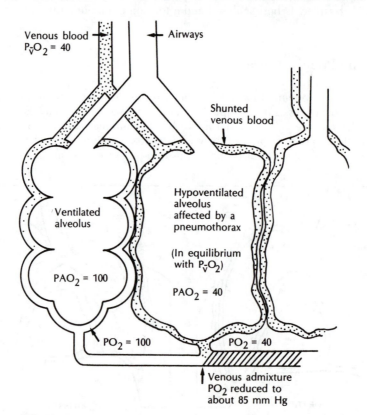

FIG 11–5.
Venous admixture in pneumothorax.

sure, and gas excapes from the pleural space through the chest wound. As gas leaves the pleural space, the mediastinum moves back toward the affected side. Because of this back-and-forth movement of the mediastinum, some gas from the normal lung may enter the collapsed lung during expiration and cause it to expand slightly. During inspiration, however, some of this "rebreathed dead-space gas" may move back into the normal lung. This paradoxical movement of gas within the lungs is known as *pendelluft*. As a result of the pendelluft, the patient hypoventilates (see Fig 11–2).

Thus, when a patient has a pneumothorax, alveolar ventilation is reduced because of lung collapse and atelectasis. Should the pneumothorax be accompanied by a sucking chest wound, alveolar ventilation may be further decreased by pendelluft.

As a result of the reduced alveolar ventilation, the patient's $\dot{V}/\dot{Q}$ ratio decreases.* This leads to intrapulmonary shunting† and venous admixture‡ (Fig 11–5). Because of the venous admixture, the Pa_{O_2} and Ca_{O_2} decrease. As this condition intensifies, the patient's oxygen level may decline to a point low enough to stimulate the peripheral chemoreceptors. Stimulation of the peripheral chemoreceptors in turn initiates an increased ventilatory rate.

OTHER POSSIBLE MECHANISMS (see page 23)
- Decreased lung compliance/increased work of breathing relationship
- Activation of the deflation reflex
- Activation of the irritant reflex
- Activation of the J receptors
- Pain/anxiety

PULMONARY FUNCTION STUDIES

LUNG VOLUME AND CAPACITY FINDINGS (see page 37)
- Decreased VC
- Decreased RV
- Decreased FRC
- Decreased TLC
- Decreased VT

INCREASED HEART RATE, CARDIAC OUTPUT, AND BLOOD PRESSURE (see page 57)

INCREASED CENTRAL VENOUS PRESSURE/DECREASED SYSTEMIC BLOOD PRESSURE (see page 57)

ARTERIAL BLOOD GASES

EARLY STAGES OF PNEUMOTHORAX
ACUTE ALVEOLAR HYPERVENTILATION WITH HYPOXEMIA (see page 48)
- Pa_{O_2}: decreased
- Pa_{CO_2}: decreased
- HCO_3^-: decreased
- pH: increased

---

*See the section on ventilation-perfusion ratio, page 16.

†See the section on pulmonary shunting, page 18.

‡See the section on venous admixture, page 19.

ADVANCED STAGES OF PNEUMOTHORAX
ACUTE VENTILATORY FAILURE WITH HYPOXEMIA (see page 52)
- Pa_{O_2}: decreased
- Pa_{CO_2}: increased
- HCO_3^-: increased
- pH: decreased

CYANOSIS (see page 16)

INCREASED CHEST DIAMETER ON THE AFFECTED SIDE

The gas that accumulates in the pleural space enhances not only the natural tendency of the lungs to collapse but also the natural tendency of the chest wall to expand. Thus, in severe pneumothorax, the chest often appears larger on the affected side. This is especially true in patients with a severe tension pneumothorax (Fig 11–6).

CHEST X-RAY FINDINGS

Ordinarily, the presence of a pneumothorax is easily identified on x-ray films in the upright posteroanterior view (Fig 11–7). A small collection of air is often visible if the exposure is made at the end of maximal expiration because the translucency of the pneumothorax is more obvious when contrasted to the density of a deflated lung.

The pneumothorax is usually seen in the upper part of the pleural cavity when the film is exposed while the patient is in the upright position. Severe adhesions, however, may limit a volume of gas to a specific portion of the pleural space. Figure

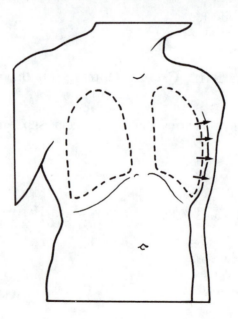

FIG 11–6.
As gas accumulates in the intrapleural space, the chest diameter increases on the affected side.

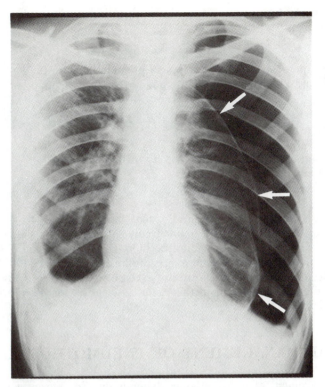

FIG 11–7.
Left-sided pneumothorax *(arrows).*

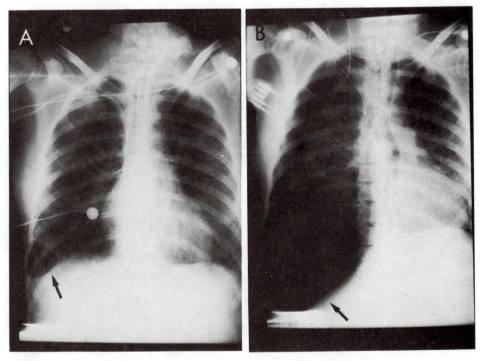

FIG 11–8.
A, development of a small tension pneumothorax in lower part of the right lung *(arrow).* **B,** the same pneumothorax 30 minutes later.

11–8,A shows the development of a tension pneumothorax in the lower part of the right lung. Figure 11–8,B shows progression of the same pneumothorax 30 minutes later.

Chest Assessment Findings

- Hyperresonant percussion note
- Diminished breath sounds
- Displaced heart sounds

As gas accumulates in the pleural space, the ratio of air to solid tissue increases. Percussion notes resonate more freely throughout the gas in the pleural space as well as in the air spaces within the lung (Fig 11–9). When this area is auscultated, however, the breath sounds are diminished, (Fig 11–10). When intrapleural gas accumulation and pressure are excessively high, the mediastinum may be forced to the unaffected side. If this is the case, heart sounds will be displaced during auscultation.

GENERAL MANAGEMENT OF PNEUMOTHORAX

The management of pneumothorax depends on the degree of lung collapse. When the pneumothorax is relatively small (15% to 20%), the patient may need only bed rest or limited physical activity. In such cases, resorption of intrapleural gas usually occurs within 30 days.

When the pneumothorax is greater than 20%, the gas should be evacuated. In less severe cases when the pneumothorax is confined to a relatively small area, air may simply be withdrawn from the pleural cavity by needle aspiration. In more se-

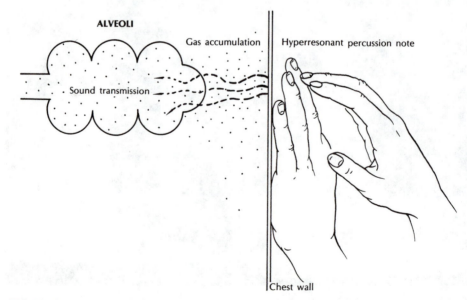

FIG 11–9.
Because the ratio of air to solid tissue increases in a pneumothorax, hyperresonant percussion notes are produced over the affected area.

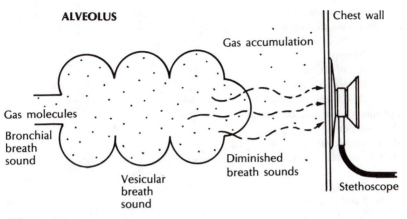

FIG 11–10.
Breath sounds diminish as gas accumulates in the intrapleural space.

rious cases, however, a chest tube attached to an underwater seal is inserted into the patient's pleural cavity. Such a tube permits evacuation of air and enhances the reexpansion and pleural adherence of the affected lung. The chest tube may or may not be attached to gentle negative suction. When negative suction is used, the negative pressure usually does not exceed -12 cm H_2O, and -5 cm H_2O is generally all that is needed. After the lung has reexpanded, the chest tube is left in place for another 24 to 48 hours.

Supplemental Oxygen

Because of the hypoxemia associated with a pneumothorax, supplemental oxygen may be required. It should be noted, however, that the hypoxemia that develops in a pneumothorax is most commonly caused by the alveolar atelectasis and capillary shunting associated with the disorder. Hypoxemia caused by capillary shunting is often refractory to oxygen therapy.

SELF-ASSESSMENT QUESTIONS

Multiple Choice
1. When gas moves between the pleural space and the atmosphere during a ventilatory cycle, the patient is said to have a/an
    I. Closed pneumothorax.
    II. Open pneumothorax.
    III. Valvular pneumothorax.
    IV. Sucking chest wound.
        a. I only.
        b. II only.
        c. III only.
        d. I and III only.
        e. II and IV only.
2. When gas enters the pleural space during inspiration but is unable to leave during expiration, the patient is said to have a/an
    I. Iatrogenic pneumothorax.
    II. Valvular pneumothorax.

    III. Tension pneumothorax.

    IV. Open pneumothorax.

       a. I only.

       b. III only.

       c. II and III only.

       d. III and IV only.

       e. II, III, and IV only.

3. A pneumothorax may be caused by

    I. Pneumonia.

    II. Tuberculosis.

    III. Chronic obstructive pulmonary disease.

    IV. Blebs.

       a. IV only.

       b. I and II only.

       c. II and III only.

       d. II, III, and IV only.

       e. I, II, III, and IV.

4. When a patient has a pneumothorax due to a sucking chest wound,

    I. Intrapleural pressure on the unaffected side increases during inspiration.

    II. The mediastinum often moves to the unaffected side during inspiration.

    III. Intrapleural pressure on the affected side often rises above the atmospheric pressure during expiration.

    IV. The mediastinum often moves to the affected side during expiration.

       a. I and IV only.

       b. I and III only.

       c. II and III only.

       d. II, III, and IV only.

       e. I, II, III, and IV.

5. The increased ventilatory rate commonly manifested in patients with pneumothorax may be due to

    I. Stimulation of the J receptors.

    II. Increased lung compliance.

    III. Increased stimulation of the Hering-Breuer reflex.

    IV. Stimulation of the irritant reflex.

       a. I and IV only.

       b. II and III only.

       c. III and IV only.

       d. II, III, and IV only.

       e. I, II, III, and IV.

6. The physician usually elects to evacuate the gas when the pneumothorax is greater than

       a. 5%.

       b. 10%.

       c. 15%.

       d. 20%.

       e. 25%.

7. When treating a pneumothorax with a chest tube and suction, the negative pressure usually does not exceed

       a. 4 cm H_2O.

       b. 6 cm H_2O.

       c. 8 cm H_2O.

       d. 10 cm H_2O.

       e. 12 cm H_2O.

8. A patient with a severe tension pneumothorax demonstrates the following:
   - I. Diminished breath sounds.
   - II. Hyperresonant percussion note.
   - III. Dull percussion notes.
   - IV. Whispered pectoriloquy.
      - a. II only.
      - b. I and II only.
      - c. III and IV only.
      - d. I, II, and IV only.
      - e. I, II, III, and IV.
9. The irritant receptors of the lung are located in the
   - I. Alveoli.
   - II. Bronchioles.
   - III. Bronchi.
   - IV. Trachea.
      - a. I only.
      - b. II only.
      - c. II and III only.
      - d. II, III, and IV only.
      - e. I, II, III, and IV.

True or False

1. A pneumothorax is always a hazard during positive pressure mechanical ventilation.   True ____   False ____
2. A pendelluft can be caused by a sucking chest wound.   True ____   False ____
3. A pneumothorax causes an increase in the patient's RV.   True ____   False ____
4. A chest tube is always accompanied by a gentle negative suction.   True ____   False ____
5. The J receptors may play a role in decreasing the patient's Pa_{CO_2} during the early stages of a tension pneumothorax.   True ____   False ____

Answers appear in Appendix XVII.

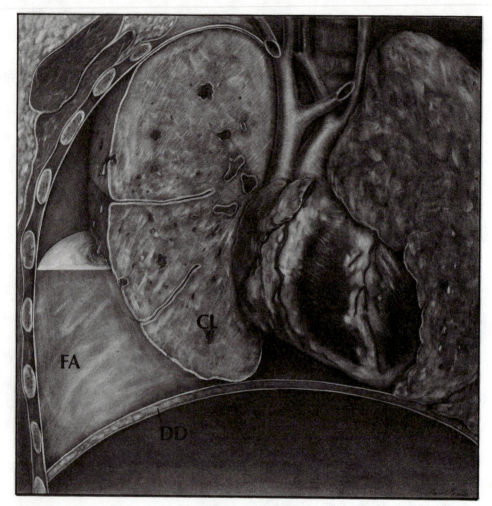

PLEURAL EFFUSION

FIG 12–1.
Right-sided pleural effusion. *FA* = fluid accumulation; *DD* = depressed diaphragm; *CL* = collapsed lung.

PLEURAL DISEASES

ANATOMIC ALTERATION OF THE LUNGS

A number of pleural diseases can cause fluid to accumulate in the pleural space, and this is called *pleural effusion* (Fig 12–1). Similarly to gas in the pleural space, fluid accumulation will separate the visceral and parietal pleura and compress the lungs. In severe cases, atelectasis will develop, the great veins may be compressed, and venous return may be diminished. Pleural effusion produces a restrictive lung disorder.

To summarize, the major pathologic or structural changes associated with pleural effusion are as follows:

- Lung compression
- Atelectasis
- Compression of the great veins and decreased venous return

ETIOLOGY

Pleural effusion may be transudative or exudative. Transudate develops when fluid from the pulmonary capillaries move into the pleural space. The fluid produced is thin and watery. It contains few blood cells and little protein. The pleural surfaces are not involved in producing the transudate.

In contrast, an exudate develops when the pleural surfaces are diseased. The fluid has a high protein content and a great deal of cellular debris. Exudate is usually caused by inflammation.

Major Causes of a Transudate

Congestive Heart Failure.—Congestive heart failure is probably the most common cause of pleural effusion. Both right- and left-heart failure can result in pleural effusion. In right-heart failure, an increase in the hydrostatic pressure in the systemic circulation can (1) increase the rate of pleural fluid formation and (2) decrease lymphatic drainage from the pleural space because of the elevated systemic venous pressure.

In left-heart failure, an increase in the hydrostatic pressures in the pulmonary circulation can (1) decrease the rate of pleural fluid absorption through the visceral

Featuring your research with a major emphasis

We have talked about the importance of getting focused on a research topic. In addition to narrowing down to a specific aspect of the substantive subject matter, your research project may also be characterized by a special methodological interest. For example, your research may focus on the conceptualization and theorization of some social phenomenon based on available information. Or you may have a special interest in measurement, and your project would accordingly have an emphasis on scale development. In some research situations you may be concerned with a major issue in sampling, such as administrative "churning" when using government agency registers as a sampling frame.

In a quantitative study, the building of a mathematical (statistical) model can be the center of investigation. Sometimes a model can be regarded as a complex hypothesis, and empirical data can be used to validate or falsify the model. A model can also be built mainly for the purposes of description, simulation, and prediction. There is an increasing interest in quantitative modeling, including structural equation modeling and Markov chain modeling, which form an important feature of contemporary social and behavioral science research.

Although research methods have typically stressed validation via hypothesis testing, attention has also been paid to discovery. In this regard, qualitative approaches have been gaining greater and greater popularity. Qualitative methods such as ethnography have been characterized by their concern with descriptive matters, or matters of particularity, in framing the research situation. Yet recent trends have indicated a growing interest in linking qualitative research with theory (Flinders & Mills, 1993). A research project emphasizing qualitative design, therefore, may also be very promising. The emergence of ethnomethodology under phenomenological philosophy and social constructionist perspective is an excellent example. Garfinkel's (1967) suggestion that people are continually trying to make sense of the life they experience and create social structure through their actions and interactions has opened a new path to social and behavioral inquiry. This accomplishment would be impossible without a thorough understanding of the research methods and a focus on the qualitative aspects of social inquiry.

pleura and (2) even cause fluid movement through the visceral pleura into the pleural space. In general, left-heart failure is more likely to produce pleural effusion than right-heart failure is.

Hepatic Hydrothorax.—Occasionally, pleural effusions can develop as a complication of hepatic cirrhosis, particularly when ascitic fluid is present. The pleural effusion in these patients is generally right-sided.

Peritoneal Dialysis.—Similarly to the pleural effusion that occurs as a result of ascites, pleural fluid may also develop as a complication of peritoneal dialysis. When the peritoneal dialysis is stopped, the pleural effusion usually disappears rapidly.

Nephrotic Syndrome.—Pleural effusion is commonly seen in patients with nephrotic syndrome. It is generally bilateral. The effusion is a result of the decreased plasma oncotic pressure that develops in this disorder.

Pulmonary Embolus.—It is estimated that between 30% and 50% of patients with pulmonary emboli develop pleural effusion. Two distinct mechanisms are responsible. First, obstruction of the pulmonary vasculature can lead to right-heart failure, which in turn can lead to pleural effusion. The second mechanism involves the increased permeability of the capillaries in the visceral pleura that develops in response to the ischemia caused by the pulmonary emboli.

Major Causes of Exudative Pleural Effusion

Malignant Pleural Effusions.—Metastatic disease of the pleura or of the mediastinal lymph nodes is the most common cause of exudative pleural effusions. Carcinoma of the lung and breast and lymphomas account for about 75% of malignant pleural effusions.

Malignant Mesotheliomas.—Malignant mesotheliomas arise from the mesothelial cells that line the pleural cavities. Individuals with chronic asbestos exposure have a much greater risk of developing this neoplasm. The pleural fluid is exudative and generally contains a mixture of normal mesothelial cells, differentiated and undifferentiated malignant mesothelial cells, and a varying number of lymphocytes and polymorphonuclear leukocytes.

Pneumonias.—As many as 40% of patients with bacterial pneumonia have an accompanying pleural effusion. Most pleural effusions associated with pneumonia resolve without any specific therapy. About 10%, however, will need some sort of therapeutic intervention. If appropriate antibiotic therapy is not instituted, bacteria invade the pleural fluid from the lung parenchyma. Eventually, pus will accumulate in the pleural cavity (empyema). Pleural effusion can also be produced by viruses, *Mycoplasma pneumoniae,* and rickettsiae, although the pleural effusions are usually small.

Tuberculosis.—Pleural effusion may develop from a rupture of a caseous tubercle into the pleural cavity. It is also possible that the inflammatory reaction that develops in tuberculosis obstructs the lymphatic pores in the parietal pleural. This in turn leads to an accumulation of protein and fluid in the pleural space. Pleural effusion due to tuberculosis is generally unilateral and small to moderate in size.

Fungal Diseases.—Patients with fungal diseases occasionally have secondary pleural effusions. Common fungal diseases that may produce a pleural effusion are histoplasmosis, coccidioidomycosis, and blastomycosis.

Pleural Effusion Due to Diseases of the Gastrointestinal Tract.—Pleural effusion is sometimes associated with diseases of the gastrointestinal tract such as pancreatic disease, subphrenic abscess, intrahepatic abscess, esophageal perforation, abdominal operations, and diaphragmatic hernia.

Pleural Effusion Due to Collagen Vascular Diseases.—Pleural effusion occasionally develops as a complication of collagen vascular diseases. Such diseases include rheumatoid pleuritis, systemic lupus erythematosus, Sjögren's syndrome, familial Mediterranean fever, and Wegener's granulomatosis.

Other Pathologic Fluids That Separate the Parietal Pleura

In addition to transudate and exudate, there are other pathologic fluids that can separate the parietal pleura.

Empyema.—The accumulation of pus in the pleural cavity is called empyema. Empyema commonly develops as a result of inflammation. Thoracentesis may confirm the diagnosis and determine the specific causative organism. The pus is usually removed by drainage.

Chylothorax.—Chylothorax (also called chylopleura) is the presence of chyle in the pleural cavity. Chyle is a milky liquid produced from the food in the small intestine during digestion. It consists mainly of fat particles in a stable emulsion. Chyle is taken up by fingerlike, intestinal lymphatics, called lacteals, and transported by the thoracic duct to the neck. From the thoracic duct, the chyle moves into the venous circulation and mixes with blood.

The presence of chyle in the pleural cavity is usually due to trauma to the neck or to a tumor occluding the thoracic duct.

Hemothorax.—The presence of blood in the pleural space is known as a hemothorax. Most of these are caused by penetrating or blunt chest trauma. An iatrogenic hemothorax may develop from trauma caused by the insertion of a central venous catheter.

Blood can gain entrance into the pleural space from trauma to the chest wall, diaphragm, lung, or mediastinum. Hemothorax may also be caused by the rupture of small blood vessels. A hematocrit should always be obtained if the pleural fluid looks like blood. A hemothorax is said to be present only when the hematocrit of the pleural fluid is at least 50% that of the peripheral blood.

OVERVIEW OF THE CARDIOPULMONARY CLINICAL MANIFESTATIONS ASSOCIATED WITH PLEURAL EFFUSION

INCREASED RESPIRATORY RATE

Several pathophysiologic mechanisms operating simultaneously may lead to an increased ventilatory rate. These are (see page 23):

- Stimulation of peripheral chemoreceptors
- Decreased lung compliance/increased work of breathing relationship
- Activation of the deflation reflex

- Activation of the irritant reflex
- Stimulation of the J receptors
- Pain/anxiety

PULMONARY FUNCTION STUDIES

LUNG VOLUME AND CAPACITY FINDINGS (see page 37)
- Decreased VC
- Decreased RV
- Decreased FRC
- Decreased TLC
- Decreased VT

INCREASED HEART RATE, CARDIAC OUTPUT, AND BLOOD PRESSURE (see page 57)

INCREASED CENTRAL VENOUS PRESSURE/DECREASED SYSTEMIC BLOOD PRESSURE (see page 57)

ARTERIAL BLOOD GASES

EARLY STAGES OF PLEURAL EFFUSION
ACUTE ALVEOLAR HYPERVENTILATION WITH HYPOXEMIA (see page 48)
- Pa_{O_2}: decreased
- Pa_{CO_2}: decreased
- HCO_3^-: decreased
- pH: increased

ADVANCED STAGES OF PLEURAL EFFUSION
ACUTE VENTILATORY FAILURE (see page 52)
- Pa_{O_2}: decreased
- Pa_{CO_2}: increased
- HCO_3^-: increased
- pH: decreased

CYANOSIS (see page 16)

CHEST PAIN/DECREASED CHEST EXPANSION (see page 70)

COUGH (DRY, NONPRODUCTIVE) (see page 58)

CHEST ASSESSMENT FINDINGS (see page 3)

- Tracheal shift
- Decreased tactile and vocal fremitus
- Dull percussion note
- Diminished breath sounds
- Displaced heart sounds

Chest X-ray Findings

- Blunting of the costophrenic angle
- Inverted diaphragm
- Mediastinum possibly shifted to the unaffected side
- Atelectasis

The diagnosis of a pleural effusion is generally based on the chest x-ray film. Pleural effusion less than 300 mL usually can not be seen on an upright chest x-ray film. In moderate pleural effusion (1,000 mL) in the upright position, an increased density usually appears at the costophrenic angle. The fluid first accumulates posteriorly in the most dependent part of the thoracic cavity, between the inferior surface of the lower lobe and the diaphragm. As the fluid volume increases, it extends upward around the anterior, lateral, and posterior thoracic walls. Interlobar fissures are sometimes highlighted as a result of fluid filling. On the typical radiogram, the lateral costophrenic angle is obliterated, and the outline of the diaphragm on the affected side is lost (Figs 12–2 and 12–3).

In severe cases, the weight of the fluid may cause the diaphragm to become inverted (concave). Clinically, this inversion is only seen in left-sided pleural effusions; the gastric air bubble is pushed downward, and the superior border of the left diaphragmatic leaf is concave. In addition, the mediastinum may be shifted to the unaffected side, and the intercostal spaces may appear widened.

Similarly to fluid accumulation, atelectasis or parenchymal infiltrates can also obliterate one or both diaphragms. Thus, when a posteroanterior or lateral chest radiograph suggests pleural effusion, additional radiographic studies are generally needed to document the presence of pleural fluid. The lateral decubitus radiogram is recommended since free fluid gravitates to the most dependent part of the pleural space (Fig 12–4).

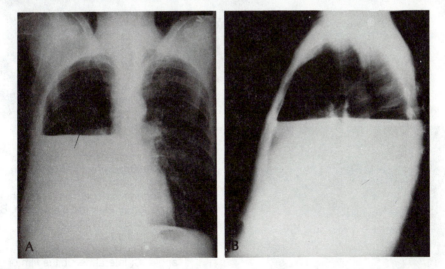

FIG 12–2.
Posteroanterior **(A)** and lateral **(B)** radiographs of a patient with a hydropneumothorax. Note that the fluid level extends throughout the length and width of the hemithorax. This hydropneumothorax followed an attempted thoracentesis in this patient with a massive right pleural effusion. (From Light RL: *Pleural Diseases.* Philadelphia, Lea & Febiger, 1983. Used by permission.)

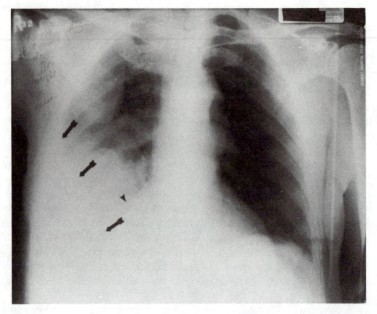

FIG 12–3.
Chest radiograph of a patient with a pulmonary abscess in the right lung, extrapleural bleed *(arrows),* and pleural effusion. (From Rau JL Jr, Pearce DJ: *Understanding Chest Radiographs.* Denver, Multi-Media Publishing Co Inc, 1984. Used by permission.)

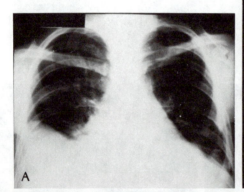

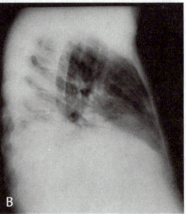

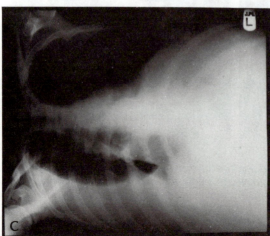

FIG 12–4.
Subpulmonic pleural effusion. **A,** posteroanterior chest radiograph demonstrating clear lateral costophrenic angles but apparent elevation of the right diaphragm. **B,** lateral chest radiograph of the same patient demonstrates a blunted posterior costophrenic angle. **C,** lateral decubitus film of this patient demonstrates large amounts of free pleural fluid. (From Light RL: *Pleural Diseases.* Philadelphia, Lea & Febiger, 1983. Used by permission.)

GENERAL MANAGEMENT OF PLEURAL EFFUSION

The management of each patient with a pleural effusion must be individualized. Questions to be asked include the following: What is the appropriate antibiotic? Should a thoracentesis be performed? Should a chest tube be inserted? Can the underlying cause be treated?

An etiologic diagnosis is necessary to appropriately treat a patient with pleural effusion. Examination of the effusion may reveal blood following trauma or surgery, pus in empyema, or milky fluid in chylothorax. The presence of blood in the pleural fluid in the absence of trauma or surgery suggests a malignant disease or pulmonary embolization.

When the cause of the pleural effusion is not readily evident, microscopic examination of pleural fluid may determine whether the effusion is a transudate or an exudate. If the fluid is a transudate, treatment is directed to the underlying problem (e.g., congestive heart failure, cirrhosis, or nephrosis). When an exudate is present, a cytologic examination may identify a malignancy. The fluid may also be examined for its biochemical makeup (e.g., protein, sugar, and various enzymes) and for the presence of bacteria.

Thoracentesis

A thoracentesis is commonly performed when pleural effusions are present. The fluid is generally analyzed for the following:

- Color
- Odor
- Red blood cell (RBC) count
- White blood cell (WBC) count with differential
- Protein
- Sugar
- Lactic dehydrogenase (LDH)
- Amylase
- pH
- Wright, Gram, and acid-fast (AFB) stains
- Aerobic, anaerobic, tuberculosis, and fungal cultures
- Cytology

Hyperinflation Techniques

Hyperinflation measures are commonly ordered to offset the alveolar consolidation and atelectasis associated with pleural effusion (see Appendix XII).

Supplemental Oxygen

Because of the hypoxemia associated with a pleural effusion, supplemental oxygen may be required. It should be noted, however, that the hypoxemia that develops in a pleural effusion is most commonly caused by the alveolar atelectasis and capillary shunting associated with the disorder. Hypoxemia caused by capillary shunting is often refractory to oxygen therapy.

SELF-ASSESSMENT QUESTIONS

Multiple Choice

1. Which of the following is/are associated with exudative effusion?
   I. Few blood cells.
   II. Inflammation.
   III. Thin and watery fluid.
   IV. Disease of the pleural surfaces.
     a. I only.
     b. II only.
     c. IV only.
     d. I and III only.
     e. II and IV only.

2. Which of the following is probably the most common cause of a transudative pleural effusion?
     a. Pulmonary embolus.
     b. Congestive heart failure.
     c. Hepatic hydrothorax.
     d. Nephrotic syndrome.
     e. Peritoneal dialysis.

3. A hemothorax is said to be present when the hematocrit of the pleural fluid is at least what percentage of the peripheral blood?
     a. 20.
     b. 30.
     c. 40.
     d. 50.
     e. 60.

4. Approximately what percentage of patients with pulmonary emboli develop pleural effusion?
     a. 0–20.
     b. 20–30.
     c. 30–50.
     d. 50–60.
     e. 60–80.

5. Which of the following is/are associated with pleural effusion?
   I. Increased RV.
   II. Decreased FRC.
   III. Increased V_T.
   IV. Decreased VC.
     a. I only.
     b. III only.
     c. I and III only.
     d. II and IV only.
     e. II, III, and IV only.

True or False

1. Chyle in the pleural cavity is commonly caused by trauma to the neck.   True _____   False _____

2. A hyperresonant percussion note is associated with a pleural effusion.   True _____   False _____

3. Left-heart failure is more likely to cause a pleural effusion than right-heart failure is.   True _____   False _____

4. The accumulation of pus in the pleural cavity is
   called empyema.   True _____   False _____
5. Pleural effusion may be caused by a gastrointestinal
   disorder.   True _____   False _____

Answers appear in Appendix XVII.

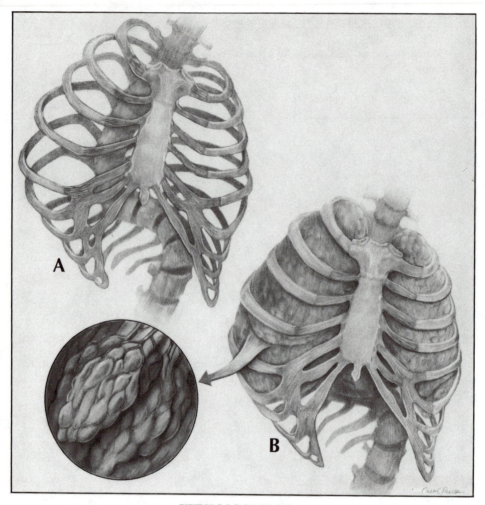

KYPHOSCOLIOSIS

FIG 13–1.
A, posterior and lateral curvature of the spine. **B,** lung compression and atelectasis *(circle inset)* caused by the thoracic deformities.

KYPHOSCOLIOSIS

ANATOMIC ALTERATIONS OF THE LUNGS

Kyphoscoliosis is a combination of two thoracic deformities that commonly appear together. *Kyphosis* is a posterior curvature of the spine (humpback), and *scoliosis* is a lateral curvature of the spine.

In severe kyphoscoliosis, the deformity of the thorax compresses the lungs and restricts alveolar expansion, which in turn causes alveolar hypoventilation and atelectasis. In addition, the patient's ability to cough and mobilize secretions may also be impaired, further causing atelectasis as secretions accumulate throughout the tracheobronchial tree. Because kyphoscoliosis involves both a posterior and lateral curvature of the spine, the thoracic contents generally twist in such a way as to cause a mediastinal shift in the same direction as the lateral curvature of the spine. Kyphoscoliosis causes a restrictive lung disorder (Fig 13–1).

To summarize, the major pathologic or structural changes of the lungs associated with kyphoscoliosis are as follows:

- Lung restriction and compression as a result of a thoracic deformity
- Mediastinal shift
- Mucus accumulation throughout the tracheobronchial tree
- Atelectasis

ETIOLOGY

Kyphoscoliosis affects approximately 10% of the U.S. population. Of this group, only about 1% have a notable deformity. The precise cause of kyphoscoliosis is unknown in about 80% to 85% of the cases. When kyphoscoliosis arises without a known cause, it is called idiopathic scoliosis. There are, however, a number of pathologic conditions known to cause kyphoscoliosis. These include congenital vertebral defects, neuromuscular disease (e.g., paralytic poliomyelitis, cerebral palsy, spinal muscular atrophy or injury), and vertebral disease.

OVERVIEW OF THE CARDIOPULMONARY CLINICAL MANIFESTATIONS ASSOCIATED WITH KYPHOSCOLIOSIS

INCREASED RESPIRATORY RATE

Several pathophysiologic mechanisms operating simultaneously may lead to an increased ventilatory rate. These are (see page 23):

CHAPTER TEN

Determining Your Plan and Preparing Your Data

The planning of your research project involves the articulation of your research questions and objectives, the establishment of your research frameworks and hypotheses, the identification and construction of your key variables and appropriate measures, the consideration of the type and structure of data to be used, the triangulation of data collection and analysis methods, and the setting of an agenda for reporting and publishing the results. Research begins when you start the planning process. A substantial part of the theoretical work should be done and be documented in the research plan. The plan is formally called a research proposal, which also lays the groundwork for your research report. Implementation of the plan mainly refers to the carrying out of data collection and analysis tasks. We will talk about data analysis in the next chapter. Here we will summarize preceding chapters in terms of submitting your research proposal, collecting the data, and preparing them for analysis.

Your research proposal

While you are going through the planning process, putting your thoughts together and writing them down will result in a research proposal. It is a good practice if you can jot it down whenever an important research idea comes to your mind. And documenting the thinking process in the form of writing a structured research proposal will give your research an important guide and thrust. In a sense, the best way to start your research is to begin your proposal writing. The research proposal is not just a useful research tool and a necessary personal

- Stimulation of peripheral chemoreceptors
- Decreased lung compliance/increased work of breathing relationship
- Activation of the deflation reflex
- Activation of the irritant reflex
- Stimulation of the J receptors
- Anxiety

PULMONARY FUNCTION STUDIES (see page 37)

LUNG VOLUME AND CAPACITY FINDINGS
- Decreased VC
- Decreased RV
- Decreased FRC
- Decreased TLC
- Decreased V_T

INCREASED HEART RATE, CARDIAC OUTPUT, AND BLOOD PRESSURE (see page 57)

ARTERIAL BLOOD GASES

EARLY STAGES OF KYPHOSCOLIOSIS
ACUTE ALVEOLAR HYPERVENTILATION WITH HYPOXEMIA (see page 48)
- Pa_{O_2}: decreased
- Pa_{CO_2}: decreased
- HCO_3^-: decreased
- pH: increased

ADVANCED STAGES OF KYPHOSCOLIOSIS
CHRONIC VENTILATORY FAILURE WITH HYPOXEMIA (see page 53)
- Pa_{O_2}: decreased
- Pa_{CO_2}: increased
- HCO_3^-: increased
- pH: normal

CYANOSIS (see page 16)

POLYCYTHEMIA, COR PULMONALE (see page 67)

- Distension of neck veins
- Enlarged and tender liver
- Peripheral edema

COUGH AND SPUTUM PRODUCTION (see page 58)

CHEST ASSESSMENT FINDINGS (see page 3)

- Increased tactile and vocal fremitus
- Dull percussion note
- Bronchial breath sounds

- Crackles/rhonchi/wheezing
- Whispered pectoriloquy

CHEST X-RAY FINDINGS

- Increased opacity
- Enlarged heart (cor pulmonale)
- Mediastinal shift
- Atelectasis

The extent of the thoracic deformity in kyphoscoliosis is demonstrated in anteroposterior and lateral x-ray films. As the alveoli collapse in kyphoscoliosis, the density of the lung increases and is revealed on the chest film as increased opacity. In severe cases, cor pulmonale may be seen. When present, a mediastinal shift is best shown on an anteroposterial chest x-ray film (Fig 13–2).

GENERAL MANAGEMENT OF KYPHOSCOLIOSIS

Bracing

When signs of kyphoscoliosis are identified early, a body brace may prevent progression of the deformity as the thoracic skeleton matures.

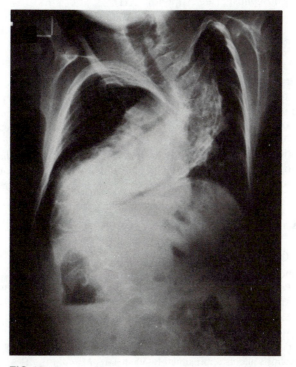

FIG 13–2.
Severe kyphoscoliosis in a 14-year-old male.

Electrical Stimulation

Electrical stimulation is an alternative to the body brace. Two methods are in use: the implantable stimulator, which is popular in Europe, and the surface electrode system. Both methods are used to strengthen the muscles that surround the spine.

Surgery

Surgery may entail fusion of the involved vertebrae or insertion of a metal brace to provide correction and stability, including the Harrington and Luque rods.

Mobilization of Bronchial Secretions

Because of the excessive mucus accumulation associated with kyphoscoliosis, a number of respiratory therapy modalities may be used to enhance the mobilization of bronchial secretions (see Appendix XI).

Hyperinflation Techniques

Hyperinflation measures are commonly ordered to offset the atelectasis associated with kyphoscoliosis (see Appendix XII).

Supplemental Oxygen

Because of the hypoxemia associated with a kyphoscoliosis, supplemental oxygen may be required. It should be noted, however, that the hypoxemia that develops in kyphoscoliosis is most commonly caused by the atelectasis and capillary shunting associated with the disorder. Hypoxemia caused by capillary shunting is often refractory to oxygen therapy.

In addition, when the patient demonstrates chronic ventilatory failure during the advanced stages of kyphoscoliosis, caution must be taken not to eliminate the patient's hypoxic drive to breathe.

SELF-ASSESSMENT QUESTIONS

Multiple Choice
1. What kind of curvature of the spine is manifested in kyphosis?
    a. Posterior.
    b. Anterior.
    c. Lateral.
    d. Medial.
    e. Posterior and lateral.
2. Kyphoscoliosis affects approximately what percentage of the U.S. population?
    a. 2.
    b. 5.

   c. 10.
   d. 15.
   e. 20.
3. Which of the following is/are associated with kyphoscoliosis?
   I. Increased FRC.
   II. Decreased VT.
   III. Increased TLC.
   IV. Decreased RV.
      a. I only.
      b. IV only.
      c. II and IV only.
      d. III and IV only.
      e. II, III, and IV only.
4. Which of the following is/are associated with kyphoscoliosis?
   I. Bronchial breath sounds.
   II. Hyperresonant percussion note.
   III. Whispered pectoriloquy.
   IV. Diminished breath sounds.
      a. I and III only.
      b. II and IV only.
      c. III and IV only.
      d. II, III, and IV only.
      e. I, II, and III only.
5. During the advanced stages of kyphoscoliosis, the patient commonly demonstrates which of the following arterial blood gas values?
   I. Increased HCO_3^-.
   II. Decreased pH.
   III. Increased Pa_{CO_2}.
   IV. Normal pH.
   V. Decreased HCO_3^-.
      a. I only.
      b. II only.
      c. III and IV only.
      d. II and V only.
      e. I, III, and IV only.

True or False

1. When kyphoscoliosis arises without a known cause, it is called idiopathic scoliosis.   True _____   False _____
2. Kyphoscoliosis is classified as an obstructive lung disorder.   True _____   False _____
3. The precise cause of kyphoscoliosis is unknown in about 80% to 85% of cases.   True _____   False _____
4. The anatomic alterations of the lungs associated with kyphoscoliosis cause a shuntlike effect.   True _____   False _____
5. Kyphoscoliosis causes the patient's RV to increase.   True _____   False _____

Answers appear in Appendix XVII.

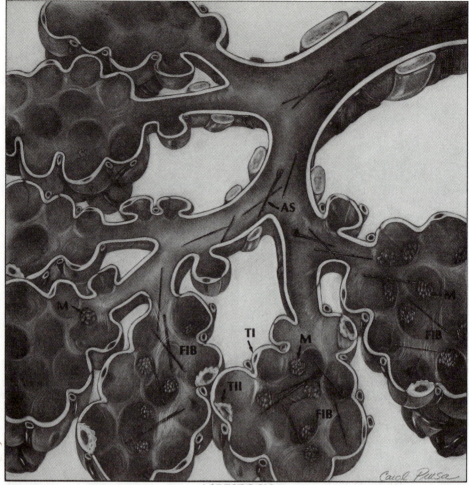

ASBESTOSIS

FIG 14–1.
Asbestosis. *M* = macrophages; *FIB* = fibrosis; *TI* = type I cell; *TII* = type II cell.

PNEUMOCONIOSIS

ANATOMIC ALTERATIONS OF THE LUNGS

Pneumoconiosis is a general term used to describe diseases of the lungs that are caused by the chronic inhalation of inorganic dusts and particulate matter, usually of occupational or environmental origin (e.g., coal dust, asbestos, silica). When inorganic dusts or particulate matter are inhaled, the smaller particles stick to the moist surfaces of the respiratory bronchioles, alveolar ducts, and alveoli.

The initial lung response is inflammation and phagocytosis by alveolar macrophages. The macrophages engulf and carry the particles to the terminal bronchioles where they are then propelled out of the lungs by the mucociliary escalator. Some particles are carried to the lymphatic vessels and then to the lymph nodes, primarily the nodes around the hilum. During excessive exposure, however, the mucociliary system becomes overwhelmed, which results in the accumulation of particles. When this happens, the dust particles become enmeshed in a network of collagen and fibrin, and the lungs stiffen (lung compliance decreases). Characteristic of pneumoconioses is the fact that the pulmonary fibrosis may continue despite the cessation of dust exposure.

Some dust particles (e.g., silica) have a toxic effect on the macrophages that ingest them. The macrophages disintegrate and release chemicals that activate successive waves of macrophages. When the newly recruited macrophages engulf the liberated dust particles, they in turn disintegrate. Some particles have the ability to penetrate the interstitial space (e.g., asbestos, coal dust, silica). As the disease progresses, the alveoli and adjacent pulmonary capillaries are destroyed and replaced by fibrous, cystlike structures. The cysts are commonly about 1.0 cm in diameter and produce a honeycomb appearance on gross examination. In severe cases, fibrotic thickening and calcification of the pleura often produce fibrocalcific pleural plaques. This pathologic process frequently extends into—or involves—the diaphragm. With some stimulants bronchogenic carcinoma may be present.

In general, the pneumoconioses produce a restrictive pulmonary disease. However, because the inorganic dusts and particular matter can also accumulate in the small airways, chronic inflammation, swelling, and bronchial constriction frequently develop. When this condition is present, clinical manifestations of airway obstruction are seen. Thus, the patient with pneumoconiosis may demonstrate a restrictive disorder, an obstructive disorder, or a combination of both.

To summarize, the major pathologic or structural changes associated with the pneumoconioses are as follows:

- Destruction of the alveoli and adjacent pulmonary capillaries
- Fibrotic thickening of the respiratory bronchioles, alveolar ducts, and alveoli
- Cystlike structures (honeycomb appearance)

- Fibrocalcific pleural plaques
- Airway obstruction caused by inflammation and bronchial constriction
- Bronchogenic carcinoma

ETIOLOGY

The etiologic determinants include (1) the size of the dust particle (only those particles between 0.3 and 0.5 μm are likely to reach in the alveoli), (2) its chemical nature, (3) its concentration, (4) the time of exposure, and (5) the individual's susceptibility to specific inorganic dusts or particulate matter. Clinically, the diagnosis of a specific cause of a pneumoconiosis may be difficult. In general, the diagnosis is based on the work history of the individual, x-ray films, and pulmonary function studies.

Some of the major causes of the pneumoconioses are covered in the subsequent sections.

Asbestosis

Exposure to asbestos causes asbestosis. Asbestos fibers are a mixture of fibrous minerals composed of hydrous silicates of magnesium, sodium, and iron in various proportions. There are two primary types, the amphiboles (crocidolite, amosite, and anthophyllite) and chrysotile (most commonly used in industry). Asbestos fibers typically range between 50 and 100 mm in length and are about 0.5 mm in diameter. The chrysotiles are characterized by having the longest and strongest fibers.

Industrial areas and commercial products associated with asbestos fibers include the following:

- Acoustic products
- Automobile undercoating
- Brake lining
- Cements
- Clutch casing
- Floor tiles
- Fire-fighting suits
- Fireproof paints
- Insulations
- Mill work
- Roofing materials
- Ropes
- Ship construction
- Steam pipe material

Asbestos fibers can often be seen within the thickened septa as brown or orange batonlike structures. The fibers characteristically stain for iron with Perl's stain. Uniform involvement of the lungs is rare. The pathologic process may only affect one lung, a lobe, or a segment of a lobe. The lower lobes are most commonly affected (Fig 14–1).

Coal Worker's Pneumoconiosis

The deposition and accumulation of large amounts of coal dust causes what is known as coal worker's pneumoconiosis (CWP). CWP is also known as *coal miner's lung, black lung, black phthisis,* and *miner's phthisis.* Miners who use cutting machines at the coal face have the greatest exposure.

Simple CWP is characterized by pinpoint nodules throughout the lungs called *coal macules* (black spots). The coal macules often develop around the first- and second-generation respiratory bronchioles and cause the adjacent alveoli to retract. This condition is called *focal emphysema.*

Complicated CWP or progressive massive fibrosis (PMF) is characterized by massive areas of fibrotic nodules greater than 1 cm. The fibrotic nodules generally appear in the peripheral regions of upper lobes and extend toward the hilum with growth. The nodules are composed of dense collagenous tissue with black pigmentation. Finally, it should be noted that coal dust by itself is chemically inert. The fibrotic changes in CWP are usually due to silica.

Silicosis

Silicosis (also called grinder's disease and quartz silicosis) is caused by the chronic inhalation of crystalline, free silica or silicon dioxide particles. Silica is the main component of more than 95% of the rocks of the earth. It is found in sandstone, quartz (beach sand is mostly quartz), flint, granite, many hard rocks, and some clays.

Simple silicosis is characterized by small rounded nodules scattered throughout the lungs. No single nodule is greater than 9 mm. Patients with simple silicosis are usually symptom free.

Complicated silicosis is characterized by nodules that coalesce and form large masses of fibrous tissues, usually in the upper lobes and perihilar regions. In severe cases, the fibrotic regions may undergo tissue necrosis and cavitate.

Occupations that may expose an individual to silica include the following:

- Tunneling
- Hard-rock mining
- Sandblasting
- Quarrying
- Stone cutting
- Grinding of pottery materials
- Foundry worker
- Ceramics worker
- Abrasives worker
- Brick maker
- Paint maker
- Polisher
- Stonecutter
- Stone driller
- Well driller

record. Since scientific research has become an institutional thing in our society, the research proposal now serves as a formal document of request for evaluation, approval, and funding. You must show, for example, that you have taken proper measures to protect the rights of human subjects, if any, that will be involved in your research project. You also need to show that your budget is reasonable, sufficient, and not inflated in view of the often tough funding situation.

We have talked about your thesis/dissertation proposal as a training tool in chapter two. In a "real" research setting, the main institutional use of a research proposal is to apply for funding. Since each funding source has its own specifications for writing a research proposal, it is crucial for you to carefully study and follow all the requirements contained in the funding source's Request for Proposal (RFP) or other guidelines. You should contact the funding source directly if you have any questions. By talking to the representatives of the funding source, you may get to know some particular expectations that are not explicitly indicated in the RFP or other guidelines. This might help you enormously with your decision about whether or not and how to invest your time in writing the proposal. To write such a proposal, special attention should be paid to your budget. Each item of spending needs to be carefully justified. This is usually determined by two factors: the amount of work involved, and the rate of spending or the amount of money needed for each unit of work required. The total amount of work should be carefully calculated in the planning of your research project with the proper division of labor. For the various kinds of labor, you should use the prevailing rates to calculate the costs. Yet for what can be considered as "prevailing," you must have an appropriate referential framework in mind. This may require you to investigate various information sources, such as looking at some related and previously successful proposals, and/or inquiring about the institutional stipulations for the payment rates. In view of the many proposals shot off by reviewers with unreasonable rates, it is worth spending time to find out what are the reasonable expectations in a particular research setting and funding process. In addition to the issue of labor rates, some budget items may be especially sensitive in a specific funding process. Such items may include spending on equipment and travel. If your project involves such costs, the guidelines for the submission of an application may contain some warnings or signals about this. If you do not have a price list handy, you may just go window shopping or make some phone calls to get some price quotes for the proposed equipment. You can also give the major airlines a call to find out the airfare for travel within a specific period and destination.

Berylliosis

Beryllium is a steel-gray, lightweight metal found in certain plastics and ceramics, rocket fuels, and x-ray tubes. As a raw ore, beryllium is not hazardous. However, when it is processed into the pure metal or one of its salts, it may cause a tissue reaction when inhaled or implanted into the skin. The acute inhalation of beryllium fumes or particles may cause a toxic or allergic pneumonitis sometimes accompanied by rhinitis, pharyngitis, and tracheobronchitis. The more complex form of berylliosis is characterized by the development of granulomas and a diffuse interstitial inflammatory reaction.

Additional causes of pneumoconiosis include the following:

- Aluminum
  - Ammunition workers
- Baritosis (barium)
  - Barite millers and miners
  - Ceramics workers
- Kaolinosis (clay)
  - Brick makers
  - Ceramics workers
  - Potters
- Siderosis (iron)
  - Welders
- Talcosis (certain talcs)
  - Ceramics workers
  - Papermakers
  - Plastics workers
  - Rubber workers

OVERVIEW OF THE CARDIOPULMONARY CLINICAL MANIFESTATIONS ASSOCIATED WITH PNEUMOCONIOSES

INCREASED RESPIRATORY RATE

Several pathophysiologic mechanisms operating simultaneously may lead to an increased ventilatory rate. These are (see page 23):

- Stimulation of peripheral chemoreceptors
- Decreased lung compliance/increased work of breathing relationship
- Stimulation of the J receptors
- Pain/anxiety

PULMONARY FUNCTION STUDIES

LUNG VOLUME AND CAPACITY FINDINGS (see page 37)
- Decreased VC
- Decreased RV
- Decreased FRC
- Decreased TLC
- Decreased V_T

EXPIRATORY MANEUVER FINDINGS (see page 38)
- Decreased FVC
- Decreased $FEF_{200-1,200}$
- Decreased $FEF_{25\%-75\%}$
- Decreased FEVT
- Decreased FEV_1/FVC ratio
- Decreased MVV
- Decreased PEFR
- Decreased $\dot{V}_{max50}$

OTHER (see page 37)
- Decreased DL_{CO}

INCREASED HEART RATE, CARDIAC OUTPUT, AND BLOOD PRESSURE (see page 57)

ARTERIAL BLOOD GASES

EARLY STAGES OF PNEUMONCONIOSIS
ACUTE ALVEOLAR HYPERVENTILATION WITH HYPOXEMIA (see page 48)
- Pa_{O_2}: decreased
- Pa_{CO_2}: decreased
- HCO_3^-: decreased
- pH: increased

ADVANCED STAGES OF PNEUMONCONIOSIS
CHRONIC VENTILATORY FAILURE WITH HYPOXEMIA (see page 53)
- Pa_{O_2}: decreased
- Pa_{CO_2}: increased
- HCO_3^-: increased
- pH: normal

CYANOSIS (see page 16)

POLYCYTHEMIA/COR PULMONALE (see page 67)

- Distension of neck veins
- Enlarged and tender liver
- Peripheral edema

DIGITAL CLUBBING (see page 70)

COUGH AND SPUTUM PRODUCTION (see page 58)

CHEST PAIN/DECREASED CHEST EXPANSION (see page 70)

PLEURAL EFFUSION (see Chapter 12)

CHEST ASSESSMENT FINDINGS (see page 3)

- Increased tactile and vocal fremitus
- Dull percussion notes

- Bronchial breath sounds
- Crackles/rhonchi/wheezes
- Pleural friction rub
- Whispered pectoriloquy

CHEST X-RAY FINDINGS

- Small rounded opacities scattered through the lungs
- Irregularly shaped opacities
- Irregular cardiac and diaphragmatic border
- Pleural plaques
- Honeycomb appearance

Because of the inflammation, tissue thickening, fibrosis, calcification, and pleural plaques, the density of the lungs progressively increases. This increased lung density resists x-ray penetration and is revealed on x-ray films as increased opacity (i.e., whiter in appearance).

Patients with simple silicosis often show small rounded opacities scattered throughout the lung. In complicated silicosis, huge densities are often seen in the upper lung fields. The hilar region may be elevated, and the lower lobes may show emphysematous changes. Another characteristic feature in a small percentage of patients with silicosis is the appearance of eggshell-like calcifications around the hilar region.

In patients with coal worker's pneumoconiosis, the rounded opacities scattered throughout the lung are smaller and less well defined than are those seen in silicosis. In general, however, the radiographic appearance of silicosis and coal worker's pneumoconiosis is very similar. When large opacities are present (greater than 1 cm), complicated coal worker's pneumoconiosis is indicated. Cavitation may also be revealed on chest x-ray films.

In patients with asbestosis, the opacity is frequently described as a clouding or "ground-glass" appearance and is particularly noted in the lower lung lobes (Fig 14–2). When there are substantial calcifications and pleural plaques in the pleural space, irregularly shaped opacities are often seen. Pleural plaques may also be seen on the superior border of the diaphragm (Fig 14–3). The inflammatory response elicited by the asbestos fibers may also produce a fuzziness and irregularity in the cardiac and diaphragmatic borders. Pleural effusion may be present in patients with asbestosis.

Finally, because several of the pneumoconioses are capable of causing cavitations and cystlike structures, a honeycomb pattern may be seen.

GENERAL MANAGEMENT OF PNEUMOCONIOSIS

Control and prevention of occupational diseases is the responsibility of the individual worker, management, the community health service, and the state and federal governments. As in all occupational diseases, prevention is the key. It involves education in protective measures, management's cooperation in supplying proper equipment and conditions, inspection and testing services provided by management and by the government, adequate medical and first-aid services at the work site, adequate hospitalization insurance and compensation, and research to provide better methods of safety.

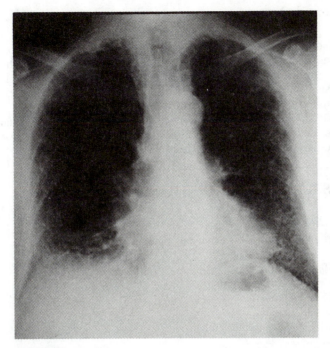

FIG 14–2.
Chest x-ray film of a patient with asbestosis.

Once the disease is established, there is no effective cure. Individuals who demonstrate suspicious clinical manifestations should be removed from any environment in which they are exposed to inorganic dusts and particulate matter. The long-term prognosis of workers who develop pneumoconiosis is poor. Treatment is directed toward symptoms of the disease.

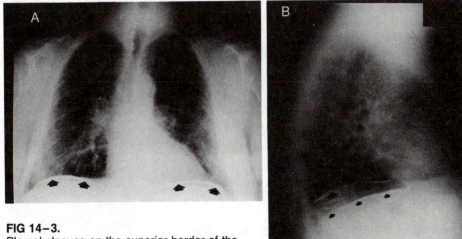

FIG 14–3.
Pleural plaques on the superior border of the diaphragm *(arrows).* **A,** anteroposterior view. **B,** lateral view.

Supplemental Oxygen

Because of the hypoxemia associated with a pneumonconiosis disorder, supplemental oxygen may be required. It should be noted, however, that the hypoxemia that develops in pneumonconiosis is most commonly caused by the alveolar thickening, fibrosis, and capillary shunting associated with the disorder. Hypoxemia caused by capillary shunting is often refractory to oxygen therapy.

In addition, when the patient demonstrates chronic ventilatory failure during the advanced stages of a pneumonconiosis disorder, caution must be taken not to eliminate the patient's hypoxic drive to breathe.

SELF-ASSESSMENT QUESTIONS

Multiple Choice

1. The length of asbestos fibers commonly ranges between
   - a. 5 and 10 mm.
   - b. 10 and 20 mm.
   - c. 15 and 25 mm.
   - d. 25 and 50 mm.
   - e. 50 and 100 mm.

2. The "J" receptors are stimulated by
   - I. Hypotension.
   - II. Lung inflation.
   - III. Hypertension.
   - IV. Lung deflation.
   - a. II only.
   - b. III only.
   - c. I and II only.
   - d. III and IV only.
   - e. I, III, and IV only.

3. When the peripheral chemoreceptors are stimulated, the patient's
   - I. Rate of breathing increases.
   - II. Heart rate decreases.
   - III. Blood pressure increases.
   - IV. Pulmonary reflex is activated.
   - a. I and II only.
   - b. I and IV only.
   - c. I, III, and IV only.
   - d. II, III, and IV only.
   - e. I, II, III, and IV.

4. The fibrotic changes that develop in coal worker's pneumonconiosis are usually due to
   - a. Barium.
   - b. Silica.
   - c. Iron.
   - d. Coal dust.
   - e. Clay.

5. As lung compliance decreases, the patient's
   - I. Ventilatory rate decreases.
   - II. Tidal volume increases.
   - III. Ventilatory rate increases.

IV. Tidal volume decreases.
V. Tidal volume remains the same.
    a. I only.
    b. I and II only.
    c. III and V only.
    d. I and V only.
    e. III and IV only.

True or False

1. Asbestosis most commonly affects the lower lung lobes.   True ____   False ____
2. Acquiring pneumoconiosis is directly related to the concentration and time an individual is exposed to the causative agent.   True ____   False ____
3. Pleural plaques are commonly associated with asbestosis.   True ____   False ____
4. Sensory nerve fibers are found in the visceral pleura.   True ____   False ____
5. Severe pneumoconiosis causes the patient's RV to increase.   True ____   False ____

Answers appear in Appendix XVII.

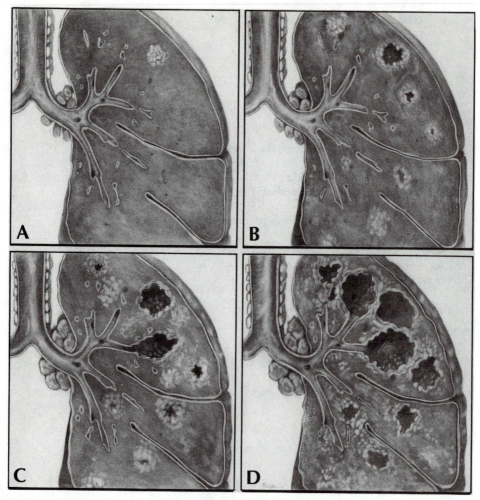

TUBERCULOSIS

FIG 15–1.
A, early primary infection. **B,** cavitation of a caseous tubercle and new primary lesions developing. **C,** further progression and development of cavitations and new primary infections. **D,** severe lung destruction caused by tuberculosis.

TUBERCULOSIS

ANATOMIC ALTERATIONS OF THE LUNGS

Tuberculosis is a chronic, bacterial infection that primarily affects the lungs, although it may occur in almost any part of the body. The disease consists of two major stages: the first stage is called the *primary infection stage* (also called primary tuberculosis) and entails the patient's first exposure to the pathogen. The second stage is called the *postprimary stage* (also called the secondary stage or reinfection tuberculosis) and is reactivation of the disease months or years after the initial infection has been controlled.

The primary infection stage begins when inhaled bacilli implant in the alveoli. As the bacilli slowly multiply (about one multiplication every 24 hours), the initial response of the lungs is an inflammatory reaction that is similar to any acute pneumonia. In other words, polymorphonuclear leukocytes and macrophages move into the infected area to engulf (but not fully kill) the bacilli. This action causes the pulmonary capillaries to dilate, the interstitium to fill with fluid, and the alveolar epithelium to swell from the edema fluid. Eventually, the alveoli become consolidated (i.e., filled with fluid, polymorphonuclear leukocytes, and macrophages). Clinically, this phase of tuberculosis coincides with a positive tuberculin reaction.

Unlike pneumonia, however, the lung tissue that surrounds the infected area slowly produces a protective cell wall that encases the bacilli to form a *granuloma*, or *tubercle*. It takes about 2 to 10 weeks for tubercles to form. During formation, the tubercles fill with necrotic tissue that resembles dry cottage cheese—hence the term *caseation*, or the forming of a caseating tubercle or a caseous granuloma.

If controlled (by the patient's immunologic defense system or by antituberculous drugs), fibrosis and calcification of the lung parenchyma ultimately replace the tubercles during the healing process. As a result of the fibrosis and calcification, the lung tissue retracts and becomes rigid. Because of the destruction, calcification, and fibrosis, distortion and dilatation of the bronchi (bronchiectasis) are commonly seen.

If uncontrolled, cavitation of the caseous tubercle develops. In severe cases, a deep tuberculous cavity may rupture and allow air and infected material to flow into the pleural space or into the bronchial tree. Pleural complications are common in tuberculosis.

It is important to note that even though the patient's immunologic defense system generally isolates and holds the bacilli in check, many of the tubercle bacilli that are imbedded within the cytoplasm of the macrophages can survive (in a dormant state) for years and even decades. Thus, a positive tuberculin reaction generally persists even after the primary infection stage has been controlled. At any time, the bacilli encased in a tubercle may escape and move into the pulmonary lymphatic system or into the blood stream and cause a postprimary infection.

In general, the bacilli that gain entrance into the blood stream usually gather and multiply in portions of the body that have a high tissue oxygen tension. The most common location is the apex of the lungs. Other oxygen-rich areas in the body include the kidneys, the end of long bones, and the brain. When a large number of bacilli are freed into the blood stream, they can produce a condition called *miliary tuberculosis*, i.e., the presence of numerous small tubercles (about the size of a pinhead) scattered throughout the body (Fig 15–1).

To summarize, the major pathologic or structural changes of the lungs associated with tuberculosis are as follows:

- Alveolar consolidation
- Alveolar-capillary destruction
- Caseating tubercles
- Cavitation
- Fibrosis and calcification of the lung parenchyma
- Distortion and dilation of the bronchi

ETIOLOGY

Tuberculosis is one of the oldest diseases known to man and still remains one of the most widespread diseases in the world. The remains of ancient skeletons from 4000 B.C. have been found with characteristic tuberculous changes. Tuberculosis was a common disease in Egypt around 1000 B.C. In early writings, the disease was most commonly called *consumption*. During the 19th century, the disease was named tuberculosis, which arose primarily from the tubercle formation described during postmortem examinations.

There are two major causative agents of tuberculosis—*Mycobacterium bovis* and *Mycobacterium tuberculosis*. The mycobacteria are slender rod-shaped, acid-fast, aerobic organisms. *Mycobacterium bovis* tuberculosis is acquired by drinking milk from infected cows and has its initial effect on the gastrointestinal tract. This form of tuberculosis has been virtually eliminated in developed countries by the pasteurization of milk and testing-control programs in cattle. Most of the tuberculosis seen today is caused by an atypical mycobacterium. The most common bacilli are called *Mycobacterium kansasii* and *Mycobacterium intracellularis*.

As already mentioned, the mycobacteria are highly aerobic and thrive best in areas of the body with high oxygen tension (e.g., the apex of the lungs). When stained, the hard outer layer of the tuberculous bacilli resist decolorization by acid or alcohol and, hence, are called acid-fast bacilli. The hard, outer coat of the tuberculosis bacillus also protects the organism against killing and digestion by phagocytes and renders the bacilli more resistant to antituberculous drugs. The tubercle bacillus is capable of surviving for months in dried sputum that is not exposed to sunlight.

The tuberculosis bacillus is most commonly acquired by inhaling infected aerosol droplets produced by the coughing, sneezing, or laughing of an individual with active tuberculosis. The bacillus may also gain entrance into the body through skin lesions, laboratory accidents (e.g., needle puncture from an infected site), or ingestion (e.g., drinking unpasteurized milk that is infected with *Mycobacterium bovis*).

Although the factors responsible for reactivation tuberculosis are not fully understood, conditions that weaken the local and systemic body defenses seem to play a major role. Such conditions include diabetes mellitus, surgery, childbirth, puberty, treatment with immunosuppressive drugs, alcoholism, nutritional deficiency, chronic debilitating disorders, and old age.

DIAGNOSIS

The most frequently used diagnostic methods for tuberculosis are the tuberculin skin test, sputum cultures, and chest x-ray studies.

The tuberculin skin test measures the delayed hypersensitivity (cell mediated, type IV) that follows exposure to the tubercle bacillus. It should be stressed, however, that a positive reaction to the skin test does not necessarily confirm that a patient has tuberculosis, only that there has been exposure to the bacillus and that cell-mediated immunity to the bacillus has developed. The most commonly used tuberculin test is the Mantoux test, which consists of an intradermal injection of a small amount of a purified protein derivative of the tuberculin bacillus. In sensitized individuals, a reaction is manifested in 48 to 72 hours. An induration (wheal) of 8 to 10 mm is considered positive. An induration of 5 to 8 mm is considered suspicious. An induration less than 5 mm is negative.

Positive Sputum

A positive sputum smear is commonly the first bacteriologic evidence of the presence of *Mycobacterium tuberculosis*. The tubercle bacilli must be stained by the acid-fast (Ziehl-Neelsen) technique. Three positive acid-fast sputum specimens are usually obtained before drug therapy is initiated. The sputum specimen should be obtained from deep in the lungs early in the morning. Saliva or nasal secretions are not acceptable.

Positive Culture

Diagnosis should be confirmed by culture. A culture is necessary to differentiate *M tuberculosis* from other acid-fast organisms. Culture results can take up to 6 to 8 weeks to obtain. Culturing also identifies drug-resistant bacilli.

OVERVIEW OF THE CARDIOPULMONARY CLINICAL MANIFESTATIONS ASSOCIATED WITH TUBERCULOSIS

INCREASED RESPIRATORY RATE

Several pathophysiologic mechanisms operating simultaneously may lead to an increased ventilatory rate. These are (see page 23):

- Stimulation of peripheral chemoreceptors
- Decreased lung compliance/increased work of breathing relationship
- Stimulation of the J receptors
- Pain/anxiety

PULMONARY FUNCTION STUDIES

LUNG VOLUME AND CAPACITY FINDINGS (see page 37)
- Decreased VC
- Decreased RV

For the student and novice researchers, what should or could be put in a proposal may still be confusing even though they have taken some research courses. Generally speaking, if you do not have a particular guideline to follow, what we have discussed so far, specifically from chapter five to chapter nine, would provide you with a framework as to what components you need to consider for your research proposal. A good proposal should clearly articulate the research questions/objectives, carefully build up the conceptual and theoretical frameworks, expressively formulate and back up the research hypotheses if any, appropriately resolve the measurement issues, and skillfully design the data structure and data collection methods. In addition, the research proposal may anticipate the main methods and equipment to be used for data analysis, as well as the major possible means for publishing the research results. Budget is not always included in your school assignment, but it is extremely important in the real research setting. For your research assignment, the use of some subheadings corresponding to these major components will help organize the proposal. In a real research setting, you must carefully follow the guidelines of the funding source or other sponsor(s).

Implementing your data collection plan

With a well-written research proposal, it should be clear what you are going to do with your data collection. In other words, you should know what information you are looking for. Here we will discuss how to make the various data collection methods work.

Mailed questionnaire survey would require you to send with the questionnaire a letter of explanation and a postage-paid, self-addressed envelope or mailing label for returning the questionnaire. These can be combined into a single mailing item through a special design, which you probably have seen at least once in examining your commercial mail in your everyday life. You should be prepared for follow-up mailings in order to increase the response rate when time permits. Since non-response usually has a negative impact on the representativeness of a random sample, you should monitor the returns and try to increase the response rate by improving the questionnaire design, choosing appropriate wording for the letter, conducting follow-up mailings, etc.

A questionnaire interview will give you a valuable experience of the dynamics of the kind of data collection process. Unless you are doing a very small-scaled

- Decreased FRC
- Decreased TLC
- Decreased V_T

INCREASED HEART RATE, CARDIAC OUTPUT, AND BLOOD PRESSURE (see page 57)

ARTERIAL BLOOD GASES

EARLY STAGES OF TUBERCULOSIS
ACUTE ALVEOLAR HYPERVENTILATION WITH HYPOXEMIA (see page 48)

- Pa_{O_2}: decreased
- Pa_{CO_2}: decreased
- HCO_3^-: decreased
- pH: increased

ADVANCED STAGES OF TUBERCULOSIS
CHRONIC VENTILATORY FAILURE WITH HYPOXEMIA (see page 53)

- Pa_{O_2}: decreased
- Pa_{CO_2}: increased
- HCO_3^-: increased
- pH: normal

CYANOSIS (see page 16)

COUGH, SPUTUM PRODUCTION, AND HEMOPTYSIS (see page 58)

CHEST PAIN/DECREASED CHEST EXPANSION (see page 70)

PLEURAL EFFUSION (see Chapter 12)

CHEST ASSESSMENT FINDINGS (see page 3)

- Increased tactile and vocal fremitus
- Dull percussion notes
- Bronchial breath sounds
- Crackles/rhonchi/wheezing
- Pleural friction rub
- Whispered pectoriloquy

CHEST X-RAY FINDINGS

- Increased opacity
- Ghon complex
- Cavitation
- Pleural effusion
- Calcification and fibrosis
- Retraction of lung segments or lobe

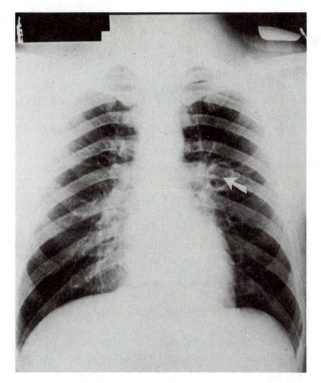

FIG 15–2.
Advanced case of tuberculosis with cavitation near the left hilar region *(arrow)*.

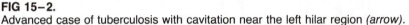

Chest radiography is most valuable in the diagnosis of pulmonary tuberculosis. During the initial primary infection stage, peripheral inflammation can be identified. As the disease progresses, the combination of lung tubercles and the involvement of the lymph nodes in the hilar region (the Ghon complex) can be seen. In severe cases, cavitations and pleural effusions can readily be seen (Fig 15–2). Healed lesions appear fibrotic or calcified. Retraction of the healed lesions or segments will also be revealed on chest x-ray films. In patients with reinfection tuberculosis of the lungs, lesions involving the apical and posterior segments of the upper lobes are often seen.

GENERAL MANAGEMENT OF TUBERCULOSIS

Specific Pharmacologic Agents Used to Treat Tuberculosis

Because the tubercle bacillus can exist in open cavitary lesions, in closed lesions, and within the cytoplasm of macrophages, a drug that may be effective in one of these environments may be ineffective in another. In addition, some of the bacilli are often drug resistant. Because of this problem, three different drugs are usually prescribed concurrently. Since there is toxicity associated with antituberculosis drugs, frequent examinations are performed to identify problems of the kidneys, liver, eyes, and ears. When the disease is identified, the patient is typically hospitalized for the first week of therapy to ensure proper compliance with the prescribed drug regimen, to monitor the patient for adverse effects, and to encourage rest and good nutrition. The standard treatment for tuberculosis today consists of several agents for a period of 6 months to a year. Drugs commonly used to treat tuberculosis are presented in the following paragraphs.

Isoniazid (INH).—This agent is considered most effective and is commonly ordered for 1 year for patients with positive skin tests. Family members are also treated during this period. Isoniazid is bacteriocidal and works to prevent the spread of active bacilli.

Rifampin (Rifadin).—This agent is bacteriocidal and is most commonly used in combination with isoniazid.

Ethambutol (Myambutol).—This is primarily a bacteriostatic drug. Tubercle bacilli become resistant to this agent quickly.

Streptomycin.—This agent is bactericidal in a neutral or alkaline medium and, because of this fact, is effective only against extracellular organisms.

Pyrazinamide (Aldinamide).—This agent is bactericidal in an acid medium and thus is effective against bacilli within the cytoplasm of the macrophages. Streptomycin and pyrazinamide are commonly used together to function as a single bactericidal agent.

Note: A common treatment regimen for tuberculosis is isoniazid, rifampin, pyrazinamide, and either ethambutol or streptomycin for 2 months and then isoniazid and rifampin for 4 months.

Supplemental Oxygen

Because of the hypoxemia associated with tuberculosis, supplemental oxygen may be required. It should be noted, however, that because of the alveolar consolidation produced by tuberculosis, capillary shunting may be present. Hypoxemia caused by capillary shunting is often refractory to oxygen therapy.

In addition, when the patient demonstrates chronic ventilatory failure during the advanced stages of tuberculosis, caution must be taken not to eliminate the patient's hypoxic drive to breathe.

SELF-ASSESSMENT QUESTIONS

Multiple Choice
1. The first stage of tuberculosis is known as
   I. Reinfection tuberculosis.
   II. Primary tuberculosis.
   III. Secondary tuberculosis.
   IV. Primary infection stage.
      a. I only.
      b. II only.
      c. III only.
      d. I and III only.
      e. II and IV only.

2. What is the protective cell wall that surrounds and encases lung tissue infected with tuberculosis?
   I. Miliary tuberculosis.
   II. Reinfection tuberculosis.
   III. Granuloma.
   IV. Tubercle.
      a. I only.
      b. III only.
      c. IV only.
      d. III and IV only.
      e. II and III only.
3. The tubercle bacillus is
   I. Highly aerobic.
   II. Acid-fast.
   III. Capable of surviving for months.
   IV. Rod shaped.
      a. I only.
      b. II only.
      c. IV only.
      d. II and III only.
      e. I, II, III, and IV.
4. At which size wheal is a tuberculin skin test considered to be positive?
      a. 4–6 mm.
      b. 6–8 mm.
      c. 8–10 mm.
      d. 10–12 mm.
      e. 12–14 mm.
5. Which of the following is considered the most effective treatment of tuberculosis?
      a. Streptomycin.
      b. Ethambutol.
      c. Isoniazid.
      d. Rifampin.
      e. Pyrazinamide.

True or False

1. Pleural space complications are common in patients with tuberculosis. True _____ False _____
2. A positive reaction to the tuberculin skin test confirms that a patient has active tuberculosis. True _____ False _____
3. Tuberculosis commonly develops in the apex of the lungs. True _____ False _____
4. The tuberculin skin test measures the delayed hypersensitivity that follows exposure to the tubercle bacillus. True _____ False _____
5. Miliary tuberculosis is a small, isolated tubercle lesion. True _____ False _____

Answers appear in Appendix XVII.

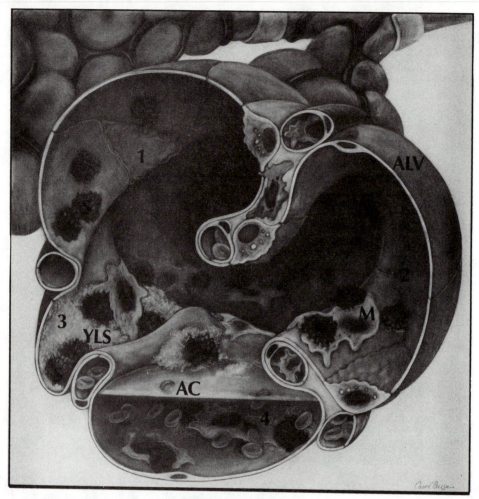

HISTOPLASMOSIS

FIG 16–1.
1, *Histoplasmosis capsulatum* spores establishing implantation in the alveolus; 2, macrophages engulfing spores; 3, macrophages and germinating spores releasing a frothy, yeastlike substance; 4, alveolar consolidation. *ALV* = alveolus; *S* = spores; *M* = macrophages; *YLS* = yeastlike substance; *AC* = alveolar consolidation.

FUNGAL DISORDERS OF THE LUNGS

ANATOMIC ALTERATIONS OF THE LUNGS

When fungal spores are inhaled, they reach the lungs and germinate. When this happens, the spores produce a frothy, yeastlike substance that leads to an inflammatory response. Polymorphonuclear leukocytes and macrophages move into the infected area and engulf the fungal spores. The pulmonary capillaries dilate, the interstitium fills with fluid, and the alveolar epithelium swells from edema fluid. Regional lymph node involvement commonly occurs during this period. Because of the inflammatory reaction, the alveoli in the infected area eventually become consolidated (Fig 16–1).

In severe cases, tissue necrosis, granulomas, and cavitations may be seen. During the healing process, fibrosis and calcification of the lung parenchyma ultimately replace the granulomas. In response to the fibrosis and calcification, the lung tissue retracts and becomes rigid. The apical and posterior segments of the upper lobes are most commonly involved. The anatomic changes of the lungs caused by fungal diseases are similar to those seen in tuberculosis.

To summarize, the major pathologic or structural changes of the lungs associated with fungal diseases of the lungs are as follows:

- Alveolar consolidation
- Alveolar-capillary destruction
- Granuloma formation
- Cavitation
- Fibrosis and calcification of the lung parenchyma

ETIOLOGY

Histoplasmosis

Histoplasmosis is the most common fungal infection in the United States. It is caused by the dimorphic fungus *Histoplasma capsulatum*. On the basis of skin testing surveys it is estimated that about 20% of the population in the United States have been infected with the disease. Cases of histoplasmosis are especially high along the major river valleys of the Midwest, e.g., Ohio, Mississippi, and Missouri.

Histoplasma capsulatum is commonly found in soils enriched with bird excreta such as the soil near chicken houses, pigeon lofts, barns, and trees where starlings and blackbirds roost. The birds themselve, however, do not carry the organism, although the *Histoplasma capsulatum* spore may be carried by bats. Generally, an individual acquires the infection by inhaling the fungal spores that are released when the soil from an infected area is disturbed, e.g., children playing in the dirt.

When the *Histoplasma capsulatum* organism reaches the alveoli, at body temperature it converts from its mycelial form (mold) to a parasitic yeast form. Depending on the individual's immune system, the disease may take on one of four forms: (1) latent asymptomatic disease, (2) self-limiting primary disease, (3) chronic histoplasmosis, or (4) disseminated infection.

Latent asymptomatic histoplasmosis is characterized by healed lesions in the lungs or hilar lymph nodes as well as a positive histoplasmin skin test.

Self-limiting primary histoplasmosis appears as a mild, febrile, respiratory infection. Early clinical manifestations include muscle and joint pains and a dry, hacking cough. Hivelike lesions (erythema multiforme) and subcutaneous nodules (erythema nodosum) may appear. During this phase of the disease, the patient's chest x-ray films generally show single or multiple infection sites.

Patients with *chronic histoplasmosis* have infiltration and cavitations of the upper lobes of one or both lungs. Clinically, this stage of the disease is similar to secondary tuberculosis and is more commonly seen in middle-aged men who also smoke. This form of histoplasmosis may be self-limiting. In some patients, however, there may be progressive destruction of lung tissue and dissemination of the infection.

Disseminated histoplasmosis may follow either primary or chronic histoplasmosis. It is most often seen in the very old or very young or in patients with abnormal immune systems. Even though the macrophages can remove the fungi from the blood stream, they are unable to kill them.

The clinical manifestations of disseminated histoplasmosis include a high-grade fever, generalized lymph node enlargement, hepatosplenomegaly, muscle wasting, anemia, leukopenia, and thrombocytopenia. The patient may be hoarse and have ulcerations of the mouth and tongue, nausea, vomiting, diarrhea, and abdominal pain. A feature of disseminated histoplasmosis may be meningitis.

The histoplasmosis skin test (similar to the tuberculosis skin test) is used to determine the presence of the organism. The presence of *Histoplasma capsulatum* causes a delayed hypersensitivity immune response. A positive finding does not tell whether the disease is recent or old. Confirmation of histoplasmosis requires culture and identification of the organism.

When the histoplasmosis organism is present, the humoral immune system responds to the acute infection by producing antibodies. Even though these antibodies are not protective, they are excellent evidence for the presence of the disease. The complement fixation test is used to show the presence of these antibodies. The presence of antibodies can also be shown with the immunodiffusion test. Both become positive 2 weeks after the general clinical manifestations of the disease.

Coccidioidomycosis

Coccidioidomycosis is caused by inhaling the spores of *Coccidioides immitis*, which are spherical cells carried by wind-borne dust particles. The disease is endemic in hot, dry regions. In the United States, it is especially prevalent in California, Arizona, Nevada, New Mexico, Texas, and Utah. About 80% of the people in the San Joaquin Valley are coccidioidin-positive. It is estimated that about 100,000 new cases occur annually. The disease is also known as California disease, desert fever, San Joaquin Valley fever, or valley fever.

When *Coccidioides immitis* spores are inhaled, they settle in the lungs, begin to germinate, and form round, thin-walled cells called spherules. The spherules, in turn, produce endospores that make more spherules (the spherule-endospore phase). The disease usually takes the form of an acute, primary self-limiting pulmonary infection with or without systemic involvement. Some cases, however, progress to a disseminated disease.

Clinical manifestations are absent in about 60% of people who have a positive skin test response. In the remaining 40%, the illness is similar to influenza. The patient may have a fever, cough, pleuritic pain, erythema multiforme, or erythema nodosum. The skin lesions are commonly accompanied by arthralgia or arthritis, especially in the ankles and knees. This condition is commonly called *"desert bumps," "desert arthritis,"* or *"desert rheumatism."*

Disseminated coccidioidomycosis occurs in about 1 out of 6,000 exposed persons. When this condition exists, there may be involvement of the lymph nodes, meninges, spleen, liver, kidney, skin, and adrenals. Death is most commonly caused by meningitis.

The diagnosis of coccidioidomycosis is made by finding spherules in the patient's sputum. Two serologic tests, the tube-precipitin (TP) test and the complement fixation (CF) test, are also useful in the diagnosis of coccidioidomycosis. An elevated CF value indicates that there is risk of dissemination. The coccidioidin skin test or the spherulin skin test can be used to determine whether the disease is present. Neither test, however, indicates whether the disease is recent or old.

Blastomycosis

Blastomycosis is caused by *Blastomyces dermatitidis*. The disease is most common in young men living in North America, particularly the southeastern and south central United States. The acute clinical manifestations resemble those of acute histoplasmosis, including fever, cough, aching of the joints and muscles, and in some cases, pleuritic pain. Unlike histoplasmosis, however, the cough is frequently productive, and the sputum is purulent. Acute pulmonary infections may either be self-limiting or progressive. Extrapulmonary lesions commonly involve the skin, bones, or prostate gland. These lesions may, in fact, be the first signs of the disease. The diagnosis of blastomycosis can be made from direct visualization of the yeast in the sputum. Culture-isolation of the fungus can also be performed.

OVERVIEW OF THE CARDIOPULMONARY CLINICAL MANIFESTATIONS ASSOCIATED WITH FUNGAL DISORDERS OF THE LUNGS

INCREASED RESPIRATORY RATE

Several pathophysiologic mechanisms operating simultaneously may lead to an increased ventilatory rate. These are (see page 23):

- Stimulation of peripheral chemoreceptors
- Decreased lung compliance/increased work of breathing relationship

- Stimulation of the J receptors
- Pain/anxiety

PULMONARY FUNCTION STUDIES

LUNG VOLUME AND CAPACITY FINDINGS (see page 37)
- Decreased VC
- Decreased RC
- Decreased FRC
- Decreased TLC
- Decreased V_T

INCREASED HEART RATE, CARDIAC OUTPUT, AND BLOOD PRESSURE (see page 57)

ARTERIAL BLOOD GASES

EARLY STAGES OF FUNGAL DISEASE
ACUTE ALVEOLAR HYPERVENTILATION WITH HYPOXEMIA (see page 48)
- Pa_{O_2}: decreased
- Pa_{CO_2}: decreased
- HCO_3^-: decreased
- pH: increased

ADVANCED STAGES OF FUNGAL DISEASE
CHRONIC VENTILATORY FAILURE WITH HYPOXEMIA (see page 53)
- Pa_{O_2}: decreased
- Pa_{CO_2}: increased
- HCO_3^-: increased
- pH: normal

CYANOSIS (see page 16)

PLEURAL EFFUSION (see Chapter 12)

COUGH, SPUTUM PRODUCTION, AND HEMOPTYSIS (see page 58)

CHEST PAIN/DECREASED CHEST EXPANSION (see page 70)

CHEST ASSESSMENT FINDINGS (see page 3)

- Increased tactile and vocal fremitus
- Dull percussion notes
- Bronchial breath sounds
- Crackles/rhonchi/wheezing
- Pleural friction rub
- Whispered pectoriloquy

CHEST X-RAY FINDINGS

- Increased opacity
- Cavitations
- Pleural effusion
- Fibrosis and calcification

   The chest radiograph changes are variable. During the early stages, localized infiltration and consolidation with or without lymph node involvement are commonly seen (Fig 16–2). Single or multiple nodules may be seen (Fig 16–3). During the advanced stages, bilateral cavitations of the apical and posterior segments of the upper lobes are often seen. In disseminated disease, a diffuse bilateral micronodular pattern is usually seen, and pleural effusion may be seen. Fibrosis and calcification of healed lesions can be identified.

GENERAL MANAGEMENT OF FUNGAL DISEASES OF THE LUNGS

Medications

Antifungal Agents.— Drugs commonly used to treat fungal diseases of the lungs are amphotericin B and ketoconazole. Amphotericin B is administered intravenously

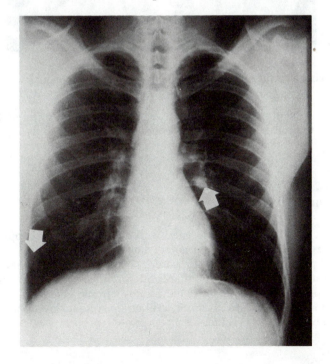

FIG 16–2.
Histoplasmosis. *Arrows* indicate a right-lung nodule and a calcified hilar lymph node in the left hilar region. (From Rau JL Jr, Pearce DJ: *Understanding Chest Radiographs.* Denver, Multi-Media Publishing Inc, 1984. Used by permission.)

interview survey, however, you may not be able to afford the time interviewing all the subjects by yourself, especially when the interviews are face-to-face. If you recruit research assistants as interviewers, you need to provide them with necessary training and guidance. If the interviewers receive pay for their work, you are better off if you are also able to motivate them by other means. The interviewers must be trained to ask the exact questions and record the exact answers. The interviewers should be able to probe for answers to minimize the number of missing values or useless answers. They should also be familiar with the questionnaire and able to clarify the meanings of the questions and avoid misunderstandings. Sometimes you need the interviewers to collect additional data by observation. The presence of an interviewer may change the way a respondent behaves and gives out his answers, however. The interviewer, therefore, should have the skill to reduce the undesirable "interviewer effect." In this regard, the appearance and demeanor of the interviewer should also be attended to. If the interview is conducted by phone, the manner with which the interviewer talks will have a great impact on the process and results.

Quality answers need quality questions. Questions asked should be relevant to your research questions and objectives, and especially the testing of your hypotheses. Questions should be logically sound (reasonable) and simple (short) enough for the respondent to be able to quickly understand and not be hard to answer.

The way of asking questions is especially important in case studies. In order to obtain detailed information as much as possible, the interview is usually unstructured so that the respondent can talk more and raise potentially important topics. The interviewer is free in asking questions, but she must have a direction and the skill to solicit the needed information. The wording of the questions, the conduct of the conversation, and the body language will all have an effect on what you will get from the interview.

When questions are delivered to a group of people rather than to an individual, you must be aware of the difference that group dynamics will make in a particular research setting. The group conversation tends to be prolonged, diversified, and harder to control. You should carefully make up each question in advance to elicit the most useful information. You should also be skillful enough to embed the predetermined focus group structure in a seemingly spontaneous and casual talk so that the data can be collected from the participants without distortion. You will usually go through several different stages of asking questions, and this may also happen in some other research settings. These stages

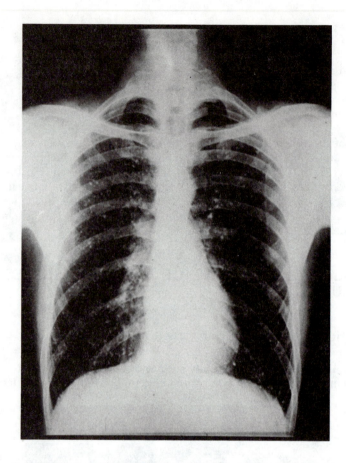

FIG 16–3.
Histoplasmosis: numerous small, round nodules scattered throughout the lungs.

(IV) and is the drug of choice in severe cases. Ketoconazole is given orally and takes up to 3 weeks to produce its effect. Ketoconazole is also used to treat progressive or disseminated fungal diseases of the lung.

Supplemental Oxygen

Because of the hypoxemia associated with fungal disorders, supplemental oxygen may be required. It should be noted, however, that because of the alveolar consolidation produced by a fungal disorder, capillary shunting may be present. Hypoxemia caused by capillary shunting is often refractory to oxygen therapy.

In addition, when the patient demonstrates chronic ventilatory failure during the advanced stages of a fungal disorder, caution must be taken not to eliminate the patient's hypoxic drive to breathe.

SELF-ASSESSMENT QUESTIONS

Multiple Choice

1. Which of the following conditions results most commonly from the ingestion of the spores of fungi?
   - a. Coccidioidomycosis.
   - b. Histoplasmosis.
   - c. San Joaquin Valley fever.
   - d. Blastomycosis.
   - e. Desert fever.

2. Cases of histoplasmosis are especially high in which of the following areas?
   - I. Arizona.
   - II. Mississippi.
   - III. Nevada.
   - IV. Texas.
     - a. II only.
     - b. IV only.
     - c. II and IV only.
     - d. II and III only.
     - e. I, III, and IV only.

3. Approximately what percentage of the population in the United States have been infected with histoplasmosis?
   - a. 5.
   - b. 10.
   - c. 15.
   - d. 20.
   - e. 25.

4. Which of the following is/are used to treat fungal diseases?
   - I. Streptomycin.
   - II. Amphotercin B.
   - III. Pencillin G.
   - IV. Ketoconazole.
     - a. I only.
     - b. II only.
     - c. IV only.
     - d. II and IV only.
     - e. I, II, and III only.

5. Which of the following forms of histoplasmosis are characterized by healed lesions in the hilar lymph nodes as well as a positive histoplasmin skin test response?
   - a. Disseminated infection.
   - b. Latent asymptomatic disease.
   - c. Chronic histoplasmosis.
   - d. Self-limiting primary disease.
   - e. None of the above.

True or False

1. *Histoplasma capsulatum* is commonly found in soils near chicken houses and pigeon lofts.   True _____   False _____

2. It is estimated that about 50,000 new cases of coccidioidomycosis occur annually.   True _____   False _____

3. Blastomycosis is also known as valley or desert fever.   True _____   False _____

4. The tube-precipitin test is used in the diagnosis of coccidioidomycosis.   True ____   False ____

5. Blastomycosis is most common in young men living in North America.   True ____   False ____

Answers appear in Appendix XVII.

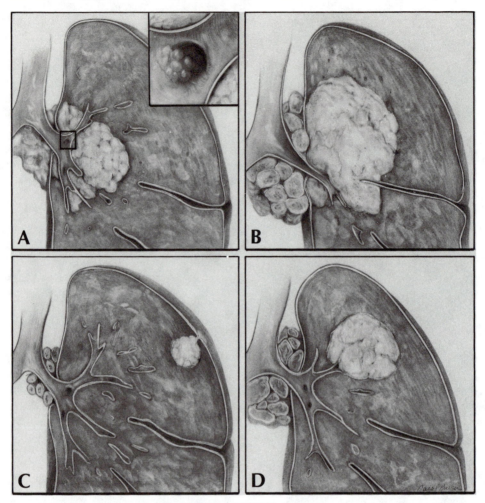

CANCER OF THE LUNG

FIG 17–1.
A, epidermoid (squamous cell) carcinoma. *Inset,* tumor projecting into a bronchus. **B,** small-cell (oat cell) carcinoma. **C,** adenocarcinoma. **D,** large-cell carcinoma.

CANCER OF THE LUNG

ANATOMIC ALTERATIONS OF THE LUNGS

Cancer is a general term that refers to abnormal new tissue growth characterized by the progressive, uncontrolled multiplication of cells. Clinically, this abnormal growth of new cells is called a *neoplasm* or *tumor*. A tumor may be localized or invasive, benign or malignant.

Benign tumors do not endanger life unless they interfere with the normal functions of other organs or affect a vital organ. They grow slowly, push aside normal tissue, but do not invade it. They are usually encapsulated, well-demarcated growths. They are not invasive or metastatic, i.e., tumor cells do not travel via the blood steam and invade or form secondary tumors in other organs.

Malignant tumors are composed of embryonic, primitive, or poorly differentiated cells. They grow in a disorganized manner and so rapidly that nutrition of the cells becomes a problem. For this reason, necrosis, ulceration, and cavitation are commonly associated with malignant tumors. They also invade surrounding tissues and are metastatic.

Although malignant changes may develop in any portion of the lung, they most commonly originate in the mucosa of the tracheobronchial tree. A tumor that originates in the bronchial mucosa is called *bronchogenic carinoma*. The terms lung cancer and bronchogenic carinoma are used interchangeably.

As a lung tumor enlarges, the surrounding bronchial airways and alveoli become irritated, inflamed, and swollen. The adjacent alveoli may fill with fluid and become consolidated or collapse. In addition, as the tumor protrudes into the tracheobronchial tree, excessive mucus production and airway obstruction commonly develops. As the surrounding blood vessels erode, blood frequently enters the tracheobronchial tree. Peripheral tumors may also invade the pleural space and impinge on the mediastinum, chest wall, ribs, or diaphragm. A secondary pleural effusion is often seen in lung cancer. A pleural effusion further compresses the lung and causes atelectasis.

To summarize, the major pathologic or structural changes associated with bronchogenic carcinoma are as follows:

- Inflammation, swelling, and destruction of the bronchial airways and alveoli
- Excessive mucus production
- Tracheobronchial tree mucus accumulation and plugging
- Compression of surrounding bronchial airways and alveoli
- Airway obstruction (either from mucus accumulation or from a tumor projecting into a bronchus)

- Atelectasis
- Alveolar consolidation
- Cavitation
- Pleural effusion (when a tumor invades the parietal pleura and mediastinum)

ETIOLOGY

There are four major types of bronchogenic tumors: (1) squamous (epidermoid) cell carcinoma, (2) small-cell (oat cell) carcinoma, (3) adenocarcinoma, and (4) large-cell carcinoma.

Squamous (Epidermoid) Cell Carcinoma

This is the most common form of bronchogenic carcinoma (about 30% to 50% of the cases). The tumor originates from the basal cells of the bronchial epithelium and grows through the epithelium before invading the surrounding tissues. The tumor grows slowly and has a late metastatic tendency. The tumor has a doubling time of about 100 days. It is commonly located in the large bronchi near the hilar region. Squamous cell tumors may be seen to project into the bronchi during bronchoscopy. In about one third of the cases, squamous cell carcinoma originates in the periphery. Cavitation with or without an air-fluid interface is seen in 10% to 20% of the cases (Fig 17–1,A).

Small-Cell (Oat Cell) Carcinoma

This form of bronchogenic carcinoma arises from the Kulchitsky (or K-type) cells in the bronchial epithelium and is commonly found near the hilar region. The tumor grows very rapidly, metastasizes early, and has a doubling time of about 30 days. Because the tumor cells are often compressed into an oval shape, this form of cancer is commonly referred to as oat cell carcinoma. Small-cell carcinoma is seen in about 20% to 25% of bronchogenic cases (Fig 17–1,B).

Adenocarcinoma

This type of bronchogenic carcinoma arises from the mucus glands of the tracheobronchial tree. In fact, the glandular configuration and the mucus production caused by this type of cancer are the pathologic features that distinguish adenocarcinoma from the other types of bronchogenic carcinoma. The growth rate and metastatic tendency of adenocarcinoma is moderate. The tumor has a doubling time of about 180 days. Adenocarcinoma is most commonly found in the peripheral portions of the lung parenchyma. Cavitation is common, although less so than with squamous or large-cell carcinoma. Adenocarcinoma is seen in about 15% to 35% of bronchogenic cases (Fig 17–1,C).

Large-Cell Carcinoma

Large-cell carcinoma may be found in either the peripheral or central regions of the lungs. Its growth rate is rapid, with an early metastatic tendency, and the tumor has a doubling time of about 100 days. Cavitation is common. Large-cell carcinoma is seen in about 15% to 35% of bronchogenic cases (Fig 17–1,D).

Bronchogenic carcinoma represents 90% to 95% percent of all the cancer types. In the United States, lung cancer is a leading cause of death among men, and it is steadily increasing in women. In fact, during the mid-1980s, the incidence of lung cancer surpassed breast cancer in women. Presently, lung cancer strikes about 130,000 persons every year. It is most commonly seen in persons between 40 and 70 years of age.

Over the past 50 years, a massive amount of evidence strongly correlates cigarette smoking with lung cancer. It is estimated that about 85% of lung cancer cases are due to cigarette smoking. Studies have shown that the risk of developing lung cancer increases directly with the number of cigarettes smoked per day. Squamous and small-cell carcinoma are strongly associated with cigarette smoking. The average male smoker is ten times more likely to develop lung cancer than is a nonsmoker. Various industrial hazards can also cause lung cancer. For example, exposure to asbestos has been recognized for years as a cause of lung cancer.

OVERVIEW OF THE CARDIOPULMONARY CLINICAL MANIFESTATIONS ASSOCIATED WITH CANCER OF THE LUNG

INCREASED RESPIRATORY RATE

Several pathophysiologic mechanisms operating simultaneously may lead to an increased ventilatory rate. These are (see page 23):

- Stimulation of peripheral chemoreceptors
- Decreased lung compliance/increased work of breathing relationship
- Stimulation of the J receptors
- Pain/anxiety

PULMONARY FUNCTION STUDIES

EXPIRATORY MANEUVER FINDINGS (see page 38)
- Decreased FVC
- Decreased $FEF_{25\%-75\%}$
- Decreased $FEF_{200-1,200}$
- Decreased FEVT
- Decreased FEV_1/FVC ratio
- Decreased MVV
- Decreased PEFR
- Decreased $\dot{V}_{max50}$

LUNG VOLUME AND CAPACITY FINDINGS (see page 37)
- Decreased VC
- Decreased RC
- Decreased FRC

- Decreased TLC
- Decreased V_T

INCREASED HEART RATE, CARDIAC OUTPUT, AND BLOOD PRESSURE (see page 57)

ARTERIAL BLOOD GASES

EARLY STAGES OF LUNG CANCER
ACUTE ALVEOLAR HYPERVENTILATION WITH HYPOXEMIA (see page 48)
- Pa_{O_2}: decreased
- Pa_{CO_2}: decreased
- HCO_3^-: decreased
- pH: increased

ADVANCED STAGES OF LUNG CANCER
ACUTE VENTILATORY FAILURE WITH HYPOXEMIA (see page 52)
- Pa_{O_2}: decreased
- Pa_{CO_2}: increased
- HCO_3^-: increased
- pH: decreased

CYANOSIS (see page 16)

COUGH, SPUTUM PRODUCTION, AND HEMOPTYSIS (see page 58)

CHEST PAIN/DECREASED CHEST EXPANSION (see page 70)

PLEURAL EFFUSION (see Chapter 12)

CHEST ASSESSMENT FINDINGS (see page 3)
- Crackles/rhonchi/wheezing

CHEST X-RAY FINDINGS

- Small, oval, coin lesion
- Large irregular mass
- Alveolar consolidation
- Atelectasis
- Pleural effusion
- Involvement of the mediastinum of the diaphragm

A routine chest x-ray film often provides the first indication or suspicion of lung cancer. Depending on how long the tumor has been growing, the chest x-ray film may show a small white nodule (called a coin lesion) or a large irregular white mass. Unfortunately, by the time a tumor is identified radiographically, regardless of its size, it is usually in the invasive stage and thus difficult to treat. The most common x-ray presentation of lung cancer is that of volume loss involving a single lobe or an individual segment within a lobe.

Because there are four major forms of lung cancer, chest x-ray film findings are quite variable. In general, squamous and small-cell carcinomas usually appear as a white mass near the hilar region, adenocarcinoma appears in the peripheral por-

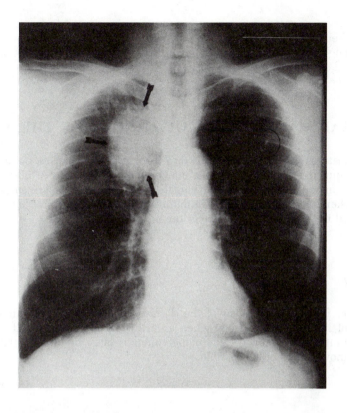

FIG 17–2.
Posteroanterior chest radiograph showing a large mass in the right upper lobe *(arrows)*. Note the nodular density in the left lung field *(circle)*. (From Rau JL Jr, Pearce DJ: *Understanding Chest Radiographs.* Denver, Multi-Media Publishing Inc, 1984. Used by permission.)

tions of the lung, and large-cell carcinoma may appear in either the peripheral or central portion of the lung. Figure 17–2 is a representative example of a bronchogenic carcinoma in the right upper lobe and a coin lesion in the left lung field. Common secondary chest x-ray findings caused by bronchial obstruction include alveolar consolidation, atelectasis, pleural effusion, and mediastinal or diaphragm involvement. The x-ray appearance of cavitation within a bronchogenic carcinoma is similar regardless of the type of cancer.

COMMON NONRESPIRATORY CLINICAL MANIFESTATIONS

- Hoarseness
- Difficulty in swallowing
- Superior vena cava syndrome

When a bronchogenic tumor invades the mediastinum, it may involve the left recurrent laryngeal nerve, the esophagus, or the superior vena cava. When the tumor involves the left recurrent laryngeal nerve, the patient's voice becomes hoarse. When the tumor compresses the esophagus, swallowing may become difficult. When a tumor invades the mediastinum and compresses the superior vena cava, blood flow to the heart from the head and upper part of the body may be inter-